Employment

Contracts

for

Healthcare

Executives

Employment Contracts for Healthcare Executives

for

Healthcare Executives

Rationale, Trends, and Samples

Fifth Edition

ACHE Management Series

Your board, staff, or clients may also benefit from this book's insight. For more information on quantity discounts, contact the Health Administration Press Marketing Manager at (312) 424-9470.

This publication is intended to provide accurate and authoritative information in regard to the subject matter covered. It is sold, or otherwise provided, with the understanding that the publisher is not engaged in rendering professional services. If professional advice or other expert assistance is required, the services of a competent professional should be sought.

The statements and opinions contained in this book are strictly those of the author(s) and do not represent the official positions of the American College of Healthcare Executives or of the Foundation of the American College of Healthcare Executives.

15 14 13 12 11   5 4 3 2

Library of Congress Cataloging-in-Publication Data
Employment contracts for healthcare executives: rationale, trends, and samples / by American College of Healthcare Executives.
    p. cm.
  ISBN 978-1-56793-339-0
  1. Hospital administrators—Employment—United States. 2. Health services administrators—Employment—United States. 3. Labor contract—United States. I. American College of Healthcare Executives.
  RA971.E48 2009
  362.11068—dc22

                    2009022414

The paper used in this publication meets the minimum requirements of American National Standard for Information Sciences—Permanence of Paper for Printed Library Materials, ANSI Z39.48-1984. ♾™

Acquisitions editor: Janet Davis; Project manager: Dojna Shearer; Book designer: Scott Miller; Composition: BookComp, Inc.; Cover designer: Deb Tremper

Health Administration Press
A division of the Foundation
   of the American College of
   Healthcare Executives
1 North Franklin Street
Suite 1700
Chicago, IL 60606-3529
(312) 424-2800

Contents

Acknowledgments

THIS FIFTH EDITION OF ACHE's publication, *Employment Contracts for Healthcare Executives: Rationale, Trends, and Samples,* is again a joint effort. Contributors include contemporary experts in executive search, healthcare management, executive compensation, healthcare law, and survey research. However, it would be a serious omission not to recognize the work of previous contributors to the earlier versions of this publication. Survey researchers obtained and analyzed the data that have enabled us to track trends. Their interviews with experts helped identify the issues that structure not only this publication but virtually all analyses of employment contracts for healthcare executives.

We are indebted to the following principal contributors for sharing their expertise and insights as we prepared this edition. Executive recruiters who reviewed content and offered new insights into developing employment contracts included Carson F. Dye, FACHE, partner, Witt/Kieffer, Toledo, Ohio; J. Daniel Ford, vice president, Furst Group, Phoenix, Arizona; Jack R. Schlosser, FACHE, managing director/practice leader, Healthcare Services, SpencerStuart, Los Angeles, California; and J. Larry Tyler, chairman and CEO, Tyler & Company, Atlanta, Georgia. Executive compensation specialists Donald C. Wegmiller, FACHE, chairman emeritus, Integrated Healthcare Strategies, Minneapolis, Minnesota; Tim Cotter, managing partner, Sullivan, Cotter and Associates, Inc., Detroit,

Michigan, and Mick Schoenberger, vice president, MSA HR Capital, a division of Integrated Healthcare Strategies, Kansas City, Missouri, provided guidance on current and evolving practices with regard to incentive compensation, benefit plans, and severance agreements. Attorneys Daniel M. Mulholland III, partner, Horty, Springer and Mattern, Pittsburgh, Pennsylvania, and Ian Donaldson, associate counsel, contributed content to update the model contracts and letters of agreement and created the model separation agreement. John A. Challenger, CEO of Challenger, Gray & Christmas, Inc., provided an expanded rationale for the importance of including outplacement services in contracts and severance agreements. Joy Lyn Bateman of Lee Hecht Harrison provided updated survey results describing the prevalence of outplacement benefits in healthcare and other sectors of the economy.

ACHE affiliates and staff also contributed to this revision. The ACHE Higher Education and Research Committee for 2007–2008 provided comments that informed both the conceptual content of the manuscript and the development of the questionnaires that collected up-to-date statistics on CEO's attitudes toward and experience with employment contracts. Committee members included William Dowling, PhD (chairman); Lloyd R. Burton, DM; Don M. Chase, FACHE; Craig A. Cordola, FACHE; Michelle D. Hereford, RN, FACHE; Andrew T. Sumner, ScD; Robert Weech-Maldonado, PhD; Marcella L. Doderer, FACHE; LTC Kevin G. LaFrance, PhD, FACHE; and Vincent W. Ng. Deborah J.Bowen, FACHE, CAE, ACHE executive vice president/COO, assisted with tireless review of multiple drafts. Reed L. Morton, PhD, FACHE, director, Healthcare Executive Career Resource Center, was the principal author of the report and benefitted greatly from the writing and editing of Douglas A. Klegon, PhD, FACHE. Also assisting with fresh content and collegial support were Peter A. Weil, PhD, FACHE, vice president, and Anne Testa, research associate from the Division of Research. Editors Eileen Lynch and Dojna Shearer managed the process of combining text, data, tables, and legal documents into this book with infinite skill and patience.

Preface

THIS FIFTH EDITION OF ACHE's *Employment Contracts for Health-care Executives* is once again the product of combined efforts. Contributors include recognized experts from executive search and outplacement, healthcare management, executive compensation, and healthcare law. This edition continues to benefit from those who contributed to the earlier editions, as they identified key issues that continue to determine the structure of this publication.

The most salient distinction between this and earlier editions is the added attention given to the perspective and the fiduciary responsibilities of the governing boards that are party to healthcare executive employment contracts. Owing to congressional interest in executive compensation at tax-exempt organizations and to measures taken by the Internal Revenue Service, particularly the reporting requirements associated with IRS Form 990, knowing and appropriately discharging the governing board's duties requires the most serious consideration. Adding this viewpoint brings into better balance consideration of the interests of the executive and the executive's employer.

Another difference between this and earlier editions is the increased treatment given to the subject of severance arrangements. The intensely challenging environment facing hospitals and their executive leadership portends growth in involuntary termination of CEOs. Severance agreements, too, must square with the IRS's expectations of reasonableness of compensation and benefits. This edition presents a model separation agreement.

Finally, this publication includes a CD that contains digital versions of the model agreements contained in the appendixes. Readers should recognize that they are only model documents. While their structure may address key issues that ought to be part of an employment contract, they do not address the unique context of the organizations in which readers may be governing or administratively leading. Considering the rationale and recommended processes presented in the text can benefit executives and board members as they approach development of an employment agreement.

Executive Summary

HEALTHCARE ORGANIZATIONS OPERATE in an increasingly challenging environment. The trend toward greater complexity and the concomitant need for senior executives with a broad range of expertise and leadership competencies have resulted in increased use of executive employment contracts. Healthcare organizations require senior managers who can confidently assume prudent risks, embrace opportunities involving significant change, and lead with decisiveness. A governing board can use executive employment contracts for the chief executive officer (CEO) and other key members of senior management to attract and retain capable and unwavering leadership during an era of change and challenge.

GROWTH IN USE OF EXECUTIVE EMPLOYMENT CONTRACTS

In 1938, the Model Contract Committee of the American College of Hospital Administrators issued a report on the value of providing an employment contract for the CEO. Current estimates suggest that approximately 60 percent of hospital CEOs have contracts. CEOs in freestanding hospitals are most likely to have formal contracts. Letters of agreement coupled with well-defined job descriptions and system policies regarding review processes and severance are more common in system hospitals. Data also indicate a growing trend of providing employment contracts to other members of senior management. After the CEO, the chief operating officer (COO) and the chief financial officer (CFO) are the executives most likely to be offered a contract.

Environmental forces that increase the complexity and risk associated with leading a healthcare organization have also contributed to the increasing prevalence of executive employment contracts. The forces discussed in this book are quality and patient safety oversight, competition, physician alignment, community benefit, transparency, and financial challenges. Spearheading organizational changes to adapt to an evolving environment increases the vulnerability of executives who may need to make controversial decisions. Boards have recognized that by providing some economic protection, executive employment contracts help provide the security that allows executives to pursue difficult decisions that may benefit the organization.

1. BENEFITS OF EXECUTIVE EMPLOYMENT CONTRACTS

Executive employment contracts benefit healthcare organizations and the executives they employ. From the organization's perspective, employment contracts for CEOs and other senior executives may positively affect four interrelated areas.

1. *Executive decision making.* The protections of an employment contract can help establish the freedom of action the CEO requires to confront politically sensitive issues. These challenges may involve status and power relationships with medical staffs and governing boards. Senior managers with employment contracts may also be

more objective about a possible change in organizational control or ownership.

2. *Governance.* An executive employment contract sets forth the employment relationship between the board and the CEO, and it can help attract and retain competent leaders. Furthermore, a contract establishes the executive's role and provides conditions for an orderly transition if termination occurs. A contract can also ensure that a well-structured, ongoing process is in place for evaluating the executive's performance. Finally, the security of a contract can augment objectivity when the board is deliberating the retention or dismissal of the CEO.

3. *Environmental adaptation.* In an environment characterized by risk and uncertainty, a contract demonstrates the board's commitment to fair treatment of the CEO in the event that a particular strategy has unforeseeable negative consequences. As such, a contract can contribute to innovation and the adoption of a long-range, strategic perspective.

4. *Symbolic value.* An executive employment contract can be a clear signal to the medical staff and other powerful community forces that the CEO has the support of the governing body and the empowerment to take prudent risks that are necessary for the organization to thrive.

Just as an executive employment contract benefits the organization, it provides the individual with four key benefits.

1. *Financial protection.* Executive employment contracts are designed to provide some financial protection in the event of termination. This protection also may check any precipitous action by the board in response to a short-term controversy or unreasonable and conflicting expectations.

2. *CEO–employer relationship.* A contract formalizes the relationship between the CEO and the organization.

Together with a formal job description, an employment contract protects the executive and the organization by clarifying major responsibilities and accountabilities.

3. *Strategy leadership.* A contract can underscore the CEO's role as the organization's principal strategist, communicating the expectation of the governing body that the CEO will accept the responsibilities of leadership and will make difficult decisions and take prudent risks on behalf of the organization.

4. *Systematic performance evaluation.* An executive employment contract can specify the parameters of an ongoing evaluation process, establishing annual objectives and priorities in conjunction with the individual's job description and defining the nature of the feedback process.

Thus, providing an executive employment contract offers mutual benefits for the organization and the individual. In its professional policy statement on the topic, "Terms of Employment for Healthcare Executives" (Appendix B), the American College of Healthcare Executives (ACHE) strongly encourages the use of contracts or formal letters of agreement for CEOs and other appropriate senior-level executives.

2. PROCESS AND ISSUES IN CONTRACT NEGOTIATIONS

Chapter 2 provides a detailed discussion of how to negotiate a contract, including (1) raising the subject, (2) using legal counsel, (3) using executive recruiters and consultants, (4) obtaining authorization, (5) developing terms for contracts, and (6) determining elements of the employment agreement. Various topics that may appear in the contract are also considered, including its term; a description of the executive's duties; compensation, including salaries, benefits, and perquisites; and the termination decision and severance arrangements.

Elements of Contracts

1. *A financial arrangement.* Executive contracts are essentially financial arrangements. The key element of a formal contract is the provision for severance compensation.

2. *No "for-cause" provisions.* Severance compensation agreements should be unambiguous. Except for a provision pertaining to intentional illegal conduct, termination agreements should contain no for-cause provisions—clauses that outline actions for which CEOs can be dismissed and denied severance compensation. Language that qualifies entitlement to severance pay raises interpretation problems and dilutes the purpose of termination arrangements.

3. *Severance range.* Ideally, the income protection the CEO receives under the termination agreement will be commensurate with the risks involved. However, as IRS Form 990 requires exempt organizations to report severance payments, it is incumbent upon governing bodies to ensure that such payments will be deemed reasonable. Executive compensation consultants have reported that prevailing severance arrangements provide CEOs with the contractual assurance of a minimum of one year's total compensation (salary plus all benefits that can be legally continued) upon termination without cause, with continued compensation for up to another six months, if needed, to find a comparable position.

4. *Outplacement services.* Executive outplacement services assist executives in transition from one leadership position to another. Outplacement services include counseling, aptitude assessments, career and second-career planning,

development of self-marketing and interviewing skills, and resume preparation. Guidance is typically offered until a suitable position is found.

5. *Preservation of the hospital's assets.* Contracts can ensure that terminated executives will not accept employment in the immediate service area for a stated period and that they will not recruit key personnel whose departure might impair the operation of the organization. Contracts can also legally bind executives to preserve the confidentiality of key information.

APPENDIXES: MODEL CONTRACTS AND BACKGROUND INFORMATION

Appendix A consists of highlights of a 2008 ACHE survey of hospital CEOs regarding their attitudes toward executive employment contracts. Two updated ACHE professional policy statements are presented in Appendix B, "Terms of Employment for Healthcare Executives," and Appendix C, "Evaluating the Performance of the Hospital or Health System CEO."

The remaining appendixes present sample contracts and letters of agreement. A long form contract, recommended for newly hired CEOs, is presented in Appendix D. A short form or letter of agreement for CEOs appears in Appendix E. Appendix F includes a recommended letter of agreement for key non-CEO executives. Finally, Appendix G includes a recommended separation agreement for CEOs.

CHAPTER 1

Growth in the Use of Executive Employment Contacts

THE EMERGENCE OF HOSPITAL CEO EMPLOYMENT CONTRACTS

Interest in executive employment contracts dates to the emergence of healthcare management as a profession. In the mid-1930s, investigators discovered that only 13 percent of hospital administrators had employment contracts (Patricia, Bacon, and Carter 1935). Despite the dearth of executive employment contracts, the Model Contract Committee of the American College of Hospital Administrators (1938) issued a report suggesting that a contract underscored the CEO's role as the hospital's ultimate authority, subject to the rules and regulations of the governing board and its ability to discharge the executive.

Although the benefits of executive employment contracts to the CEO and the organization were recognized early on, the use of contracts remained limited into the 1980s. Since that time, the American College of Healthcare Executives (ACHE) and the American Hospital Association (AHA) have conducted a variety of studies on hospital leadership and governance that demonstrate a growing reliance on executive employment contracts.

During this period, the increase in hospital executive employment contracts was dramatic. Only 22 percent of hospital CEOs reported having employment contracts in a 1984 study (American College of Hospital Administrators 1984). One year later, another study showed that one-third of responding hospital CEOs had employment contracts (American College of Hospital Administrators 1985). In 1989 the AHA conducted a study of governance in hospitals and discovered that 43 percent of hospital chief executives had contracts (Alexander 1999).

ACHE, AHA, the American Medical Association (AMA), and Ernst & Young conducted Phase I of the Partnership Study in 1992 to examine the roles and working relationships among hospital leaders—CEOs, board chairs, and elected leaders of medical staffs. The study was broadly representative of CEOs of nonprofit and state and local governmental hospitals providing short-term general medical and surgical care. The results showed that 46 percent of hospital CEOs had contracts (ACHE et al. 1993).

In 1997, the AHA repeated the earlier governance study and revealed that the percentage of hospital chief executives with employment contracts had climbed to 59 percent overall, rising as high as 64 percent among CEOs of nonprofit hospitals (Alexander et al. 1999). In 1999, a smaller-scale survey of ACHE's CEO Circle found that 67 percent of responding CEOs had employment contracts (ACHE 1999). In ACHE's most recent survey (spring 2008) of a sample of its hospital CEO members, 56 percent of the respondents indicated they had active employment contracts (ACHE 2008a).

VARIATION IN THE USE OF HOSPITAL CEO EXECUTIVE EMPLOYMENT CONTRACTS

Since the founding of ACHE and the emergence of the profession of hospital management, executive employment contracts have become more prevalent, increasing from 13 percent in the mid-1930s to approximately 60 percent by the end of the 1990s. Most of the growth has occurred since the mid-1980s, the beginning of the diagnostic related groups (DRG) era.

Exhibit 1.1 Percent of Hospitals Offering a CEO Employment Contract: Freestanding Versus System Hospitals

	1989	1997	2008
Freestanding	46%	63%	75%
System	36%	48%	32%
All Hospitals	43%	59%	56%

SOURCES: Alexander, J. 1999. *The Changing Character of Hospital Governance.* Chicago: The Health Research and Educational Trust, 13.

Alexander, J., B. Weiner, R. Bogue, and J. Isaacs. 1999. *Hospital Governance Trends.* Unpublished manuscript.

American College of Healthcare Executives. 2008a. *CEO's Attitudes About Contracts for Themselves and Their Management Teams.* CEO Circle White Paper. Chicago: ACHE.

While the increase in executive employment contracts has been significant, it has not been uniform across all settings. A higher proportion of CEOs in freestanding hospitals have contracts compared with CEOs in system hospitals. Exhibit 1.1 compares results from three time periods for freestanding versus system hospitals.

As Exhibit 1.1 indicates, the gap appears to be widening. System hospitals may be relying more on well-defined job descriptions and review processes, combined with severance agreements, than on formal employment contracts.

The 2008 ACHE survey of hospital CEOs also found regional differences in the use of contracts, with 73 percent of CEOs in the Northeast having contracts compared with only 47 percent of CEOs in the South. However, comparisons by hospital size or size of place (rural, small city, large city, metropolitan areas) revealed few differences (ACHE 2008a).

Personal attributes were shown to have some relationship to having a contract. For example, while 51 percent of CEOs under age 50 had a contract, 60 percent of CEOs over age 60 said they had one. Also, while 47 percent of women had a contract, 58 percent of men reported having one.

THE EFFECT OF EXECUTIVE EMPLOYMENT CONTRACTS ON SEVERANCE AGREEMENTS

The use of severance agreements has increased along with the growth in executive employment contracts. In a 2001 interview, Donald C. Wegmiller, FACHE (2001a), who is currently chairman emeritus of Integrated Healthcare Strategies in Minneapolis, indicated that

> severance agreements have become increasingly prevalent in health care. They are provided either through a severance policy that applies to all executives or through a severance agreement that applies individually to an executive. Most CEO employment agreements spell out the severance benefits. The most common severance period is two years for a CEO and lesser periods for other executive positions. Some organizations provide severance with a base amount plus one month's salary per year of service.

Those hospitals that offered contracts also provided severance pay for twice as long as hospitals that did not. The median length of severance pay in 1992 was a year for hospitals offering contracts, compared with six months for those that did not offer contracts (ACHE et al. 1993). By 2005, the duration of severance payments for senior executives had changed. Outplacement firm Lee Hecht Harrison conducted a study of severance and separation benefits covering 16 industry groups including healthcare. It reported that unlike other employee levels, C-suite severance is commonly based on a negotiated employment agreement rather than being determined by years of service (Lee Hecht Harrison 2005).

PREVALENCE OF EMPLOYMENT CONTRACTS AMONG NON-CEO EXECUTIVES

Employment contracts are being provided to top managers other than CEOs with increasing frequency. A 1994 study found that 9 percent of acute-care hospitals offered contracts to CFOs, 7 percent offered them to COOs, and 5 percent offered them to senior and other vice presidents (AHA et al. 1994).

Results from ACHE's 2008 study indicate the extent to which such employment contracts have increased. Hospitals whose CEOs had contracts also offered contracts to 33 percent of CFOs, 26 percent of COOs, 19 percent of chief nursing officers (CNOs), 17 percent of chief medical officers (CMOs), and 10 percent of chief information officers (CIOs). Additionally, hospitals offered contracts to 18 percent of other senior executives. However, 56 percent of the respondents stated that contracts for non-CEOs are not needed as long as there is a clear and fair policy on severance. It is not unusual for hospital executives other than CEOs to receive letters of agreement addressing severance benefits if they request them (Franck 2000; Tyler 2000).

HEALTHCARE TRENDS AFFECTING THE USE OF EMPLOYMENT CONTRACTS

Healthcare organizations operate in an increasingly challenging environment. Leading an organization to success is difficult and fraught with risk. Under such conditions, an executive employment contract can attract and retain an effective CEO and empower him or her to implement change and undertake reasonable risk.

As the complexity of healthcare organizations increases, so does the need for senior executives with a broad range of expertise and leadership competencies. The Institute of Medicine's (IOM) landmark report, *To Err Is Human: Building a Safer Health System*, issued in November 1999, was a clear indication that CEOs needed to take on new responsibilities to ensure quality. It may seem that healthcare providers face only one constant: pressure to provide higher-quality, more efficient healthcare services while resources remain constrained.

If any vision has driven a national approach to healthcare policy during this period, it is one of a healthcare market made efficient by consumer choice. Underlying this approach are new delivery alternatives, new information consumers can use to compare providers, and new payment mechanisms, such as high-deductible plans paired with health savings accounts.

The result is that hospitals and health systems now face more rugged operational and competitive landscapes. Operational challenges include critical human resource shortages, strained physician relationships, financial pressures, and demands for greater governance accountability and transparency. Add to these competition from physician-owned specialty hospitals, retail primary care clinics, and freestanding emergency care and surgical centers, and it becomes clear that leading a provider organization is not for the faint hearted.

The challenges of the healthcare landscape directly relate to the increased adoption of executive employment contracts. Effective executives respond to serious environmental threats by pursuing opportunities that may introduce disruptive change. They must propose and execute long-term strategic initiatives that can expose their organizations to unknown market and financial risks. Simultaneously, the executive may need to address internal resistance. Such situations demand a senior management team whose members can confidently assume prudent risks, embrace opportunities involving significant change, and lead with decisiveness. Contracts for chief executives and other key managers are one tool that governing boards can use to ensure capable and unwavering leadership during an era of change and challenge. Likewise, the governing board that seeks a new chief executive with proven leadership capability should recognize that offering an employment contract is a virtual necessity in competing for top talent.

Executive compensation specialist Bernard Schaeffer has suggested that the global forces affecting healthcare could account for the growing prevalence of contracts. "The many societal, political, technological, and economic pressures that have transformed the way institutional healthcare is organized and delivered in this country are responsible for acceleration in the trend toward contracts for health care CEOs" (Schaeffer 1989). These pressures have increased the risk to and vulnerability of healthcare executives, who often must make difficult and controversial decisions to deal with environmental changes.

Continuous and stressful change and its attendant controversies naturally exact a toll on the stamina of healthcare leaders. In a 2008 monograph concerning hospital board–CEO relationships, the AHA Center for Healthcare Governance disclosed an alarming trend: A significant percentage of hospital presidents and CEOs are stepping down from their positions well before the age of 65 (Cohen 2008). This trend has also been noted in discussions with executive compensation expert Donald Wegmiller, FACHE, of Integrated Healthcare Strategies (Wegmiller 2001a). Ken Cohen, author of the AHA monograph, suggests some of the factors influencing CEOs' decisions to retire early: "Many of them are tired and frustrated by dealing with medical staff issues; others are being challenged and discouraged after physicians have circumvented them and complained directly to the board. Still others want to improve the quality of their lives and are no longer willing to make the sacrifices required of these positions" (Cohen 2008, 5).

The same pressures affecting the executive leadership of healthcare organizations have also gradually changed the nature of governing boards. Not long ago, discussions of board responsibilities focused on strengthening their fundraising role. Boards have since begun to understand their joint responsibilities with the CEO for clinical quality and patient safety, the delivery of needed services, the competitiveness of the hospital, and the operation of the organization according to sound business principles.

In the 1997 AHA Hospital and Health System Governance Survey, 67 percent of respondents considered financial/business acumen to be a critical criterion for hospital board member selection, while 14 percent named fundraising as a critical criterion (Bogue et al. 1997). Additional data emerged in the 2008 AHA Center for Healthcare Governance's monograph describing best practices for developing sound board–CEO relationships. The research conducted for that monograph revealed "that boards are showing an increasingly greater focus on quality and that finance is now regarded as one of several key metrics, rather than the only or most important measure of success" (Cohen 2008, 12). This finding suggests that board leaders now recognize that the governing body of a healthcare organization is legally accountable for the quality of all elements of patient care.

In the case of nonprofit hospitals and health systems, the board is also responsible for ensuring that the organization fulfills its charitable purpose. Boards must clearly demonstrate appropriate levels of community benefit, thus justifying their organizations' tax status. Community benefit has become a multifaceted concept, including increased levels of care for patients lacking financial resources and involving assessments of executive compensation and the nature of oversight by the organization's board. As a consequence, the board is responsible for ensuring that high quality standards and charitable purpose are maintained through an internal system of organization and management. IRS Form 990 was revised in 2008 to include questions on governance and executive pay and perquisites. Beginning in 2009, hospitals must disclose, in detail, information on levels of charity care and other subsidized aid to their communities (Evans 2008a).

Ultimately, the CEO and the management team, together with the board, must be responsible to the expectations of the organization's constituencies, which include patients and their families, providers, employers, insurers, and governmental agencies. This requires skillful innovation and constant adaptation to a changing and challenging environment. Successfully adapting, which corporate transformation expert David Nadler (1964) calls "organizational frame bending," is extraordinarily time consuming and risky for senior management.

The dilemma here is that investment of time by the senior team is needed, and yet this may cut into the time that the team needs in its role as leader of the rest of the organization. This may lead to charges that the senior team is too insular, too inward looking, too absorbed in its own processes. (Nadler 1964)

Healthcare organizations that disregard the turbulent environment and fail to adapt are unlikely to endure. An effective hospital chief executive must be able to lead successful adaptation, and the governing board must provide that executive with the clarity and security an employment contract can offer.

Examining key changes that have made the hospital CEO's role more challenging sheds light on why employment contracts have become a virtual requirement for employment. A review of recent environmental pressures can further clarify why employment contracts are developing some unprecedented provisions and how contracts may protect the organization as well as the executive.

Quality and Patient Safety Oversight

Providing safe, high-quality patient care always has been a focus of healthcare executives. However, quality of care was frequently ensured by the organized medical staff structure without a great deal of CEO or board involvement. When the IOM issued *To Err Is Human: Building a Safer Health System* in November 1999, it became apparent that patient safety issues were more prevalent than previously assumed. The report laid out a comprehensive strategy by which government, healthcare providers, industry, and consumers could reduce preventable medical errors.

The IOM (2008) report noted that the majority of medical errors result not from individual recklessness or incompetency, but as a result of "faulty systems, processes and conditions that lead people to make mistakes or fail to prevent them. . . . Thus, mistakes can best be prevented by designing the health system at all levels to make it safer—to make it harder for people to do something wrong and easier for them to do it right." To improve quality and eliminate errors, an organization's executive leadership and board must guide an organizational culture dedicated to improvement, focusing resources on the structures, processes, and monitoring systems that will ensure that patients receive the care they need without risk of harm.

The emergence of clinical quality and patient safety as core oversight functions of the CEO and board introduced new challenges and responsibilities but also risks, including challenges from medical staff members regarding the validity of quality measures and the CEO's qualifications (Dye 2008), the market risk of increased public scrutiny, the financial risk of pay-for-performance, and the avoidance of "never events" (serious reportable events, such as wrong-site surgery, that never should occur).

The Changing Nature of Competition: Concentration of Power

In the 1990s, advocates of a more competitive healthcare marketplace saw the growth of managed care and the rise of integrated delivery networks as key forces in increasing competition and achieving a more effective and efficient healthcare delivery system. However, both systems have undergone change that has produced waves of consolidations. As a result, the insurance and the provider markets have become more concentrated.

For example, in 1990, 33 million HMO enrollees were spread among 572 HMOs. By 2006, HMO enrollment had grown to 73 million individuals in 541 plans (ACHE 2008c). The growth in average plan size was accompanied by a decline in provider-owned plans, as those plans were acquired by larger competitors seeking to increase their membership base and extend their geographic reach (Vesely 2008b).

On the provider side, the total number of community hospitals declined from 5,420 in 1990 to 4,947 in 2006 (ACHE 2008c), while the number of system hospitals grew from 2,542 in 2000 to 2,669 in 2004 (*Modern Healthcare* 2005). *Modern Healthcare* reported that in 2007, hospitals and systems concluded 103 deals affecting 214 hospitals; most were acquisitions by for-profit chains. Looking to the future, however, *Modern Healthcare* predicted that large not-for-profits would become the dominant strategic acquirers, "snapping up a hospital here and there to keep another large, healthy system out of their market or to build market share to win more leverage with payers" (Evans and Galloro 2008, 21). Irving Levin Associates reported that despite the 2008 capital market crisis, merger and acquisition activity in the healthcare sector is still strong. The explanation is that the underlying reasons to pursue healthcare mergers and acquisitions remain firmly in place: to consolidate fragmented providers, to achieve economies of scale, and to meet the increasing demand for services and new technologies (Irving Levin Associates 2009).

As a consequence, negotiating power is more concentrated on both sides of the healthcare marketplace. This has led to greater risks and the potential for intense conflicts, such as the four-year battle between Advocate Health Care, a hospital network in the Chicago area, and UnitedHealthcare, an insurer. In this case, Advocate terminated its contract with UnitedHealthcare at the end of 2003, affecting 40,000 Advocate patients who had coverage with the insurer (Knowles 2003; *Business Wire* 2007). Such high-stakes negotiating to maintain or enhance the organization's strategic integrity exemplifies the prudent risk taking an employment agreement supports. As Jack Schlosser, FACHE (2008), observed,

> Weathering one of these storms with the CEO at the helm requires a governance team to have the courage of conviction. That courage may be bolstered knowing that it will be costly to toss overboard the CEO under contract and then face the challenge of finding a next CEO who may also expect the security of an employment contract.

Physician Alignment and Complexity Risk

Hospital–physician relations have been an enduring challenge for healthcare CEOs. However, the CEO who strives for harmonious relations with a medical staff likely exposes the organization to substantial "complexity risk." The CEO's relations with individual physicians, physician groups, and the medical staff as a whole may require a knife-edge balance between order and chaos to pursue essential strategic initiatives. Three forces that have introduced unpredictability and uncertainty are (1) physician requests for payment for service to the hospital, (2) competition with physician-owned facilities and equipment, and (3) changing medical staff structures and leadership (Kaufman 2008).

Today, CEOs follow new models for employing primary care and specialized physicians and surgeons. Sometimes it is necessary to pay physicians to be on call. Sometimes CEOs need to keep physicians from becoming competitors (e.g., by employing cardiologists to head off the entry of a physician-owned hospital entity, such as MedCath, into the market). And some physicians prefer being employed by a hospital to running their own practice. Younger physicians in particular tend to value the work/life balance typically associated with hospital employment.

Physician-owned facilities can be especially vexing for hospital CEOs. Kevin H. Mosser, MD, senior vice president at WellSpan Health and president of Gettysburg Hospital, remarks that these facilities, such as outpatient surgery, imaging, physical therapy, or laboratory services, are attractive to physicians in the face of escalating cost pressures on traditional practices and reduced reimbursement. But these activities often involve services that have been traditional profit sources for hospitals. As David Ollier Weber (2006, 9) points out, "that's very threatening to hospitals, because those things pay for all the rest of the stuff we do."

Employment and other financial relationships with physicians produce new financial risks and rewards for a healthcare organization. Having mixed medical staff models (employed and independent physicians) makes decision making more complex, particularly as it affects resource allocation. Employing physicians adds payroll expense that must be justified by productivity. Also, employed doctors are not like other employees. They may want a greater voice in more decisions and to be treated more like partners, only accepting mentoring and management from other physicians. However, if other medical staff members perceive favoritism in the treatment of employed physicians, they may become resentful and seek competitive options.

Governmental Expectations Regarding Compensation and Community Benefit

The spillover effect of the Sarbanes-Oxley legislation may influence healthcare executive employment contracts. Although Sarbanes-Oxley was developed to apply to investor-owned organizations, the legislative intent, especially in terms of transparency, is directly and indirectly affecting nonprofit healthcare organizations.

The indirect effect arises from the sensitivity of hospital board members who lead businesses that *are* directly affected by Sarbanes-Oxley requirements. They may have elevated expectations of transparency based on contending daily with that legislation's requirements. More direct influence stems from federal activity that is consonant with the intent of Sarbanes-Oxley. These efforts include work by the U.S. General Accountability Office; the U.S. Senate Finance Committee, on which Senator Charles Grassley has served as ranking member; and the IRS. While the GAO focused on the executive compensation policies and practices of nonprofit health systems, Senator Grassley's concern extended to uncompensated care and community benefits provided by nonprofit hospitals. The IRS, through "soft audits" and a "Compliance Check Questionnaire" that addressed hospital operations and governance, explored executive compensation practices at tax-exempt organizations (Integrated Healthcare Strategies 2007).

The IRS developed a new Form 990 for nonprofit organizations, to be completed beginning in fiscal year 2009. It includes new governance questions about the composition and independence of the board and about practices such as documentation of committee actions, approval of compensation, and review of Form 990 itself. A new Schedule H for nonprofit hospitals requires a description of charity care and other community benefits provided, community-building activities, bad debt, Medicare and collection practices, and transactions with management companies and joint ventures (Kastel 2008). Section J explores specific types of compensation and perquisites and requires a description of the processes for approving executive compensation.

Hospital boards will now need to have proper procedures in place for establishing a "rebuttable presumption of reasonableness" regarding executive compensation (Miller 2001). These include (1) advance approval of the compensation arrangement by an authorized body free of any conflict of interest, (2) obtaining and relying on appropriate comparability data, and (3) adequate documentation of the basis for the compensation determination concurrent with making the decision.

Intermediate sanctions may be imposed on any disqualified person who receives an excess benefit and on each organization manager who approves an excess benefit. If excess benefit is found, the disqualified person must reimburse the organization and faces interest and excise penalties. Board members are considered organizational managers, so they also may be subject to fines (Independent Sector 2002). Thus, for the board, a well-designed executive employment contract can specify evaluation processes that provide some measure of protection.

Public Expectations for Transparency

The demand for greater transparency by government, business, and consumer advocates/activists is another source of tension for hospital

CEOs. Transparency stakeholders are requesting or requiring information on quality, finances, executive compensation, and community benefit. These data can be used to advance the positions of those who support the organization and of those who wish to be detractors.

The media's role in relation to the issue of transparency is increasing. Investigative reports may produce negative publicity when reporters fail to take a balanced approach to discussing the challenges of meeting complex and conflicting demands. Since the previous edition of this book was published, single-purpose blogs and websites have emerged. These media compound potential problems with a community's perception of healthcare, hospitals, and CEOs. Sorting out opinion from fact is not easy and is especially challenging when biased sources exist.

To give an example of the increased scrutiny that electronic media allow, one website, WhereTheMoneyGoes.com, has highlighted perquisites, such as club memberships, that specific CEOs have received. Traditional media also increasingly treat hospital profits, CEO compensation, and levels of community service with a critical eye. Rather than touting their organization's role as a community resource, CEOs are likely to be required to defend their performance in a difficult environment.

Given an environment that is charged by perception, emotion, and politics, a CEO must have reasonable protection from short-term reactions to criticism. Such protections, however, should only exist so long as the CEO's behavior conforms to appropriate ethical and legal standards. Given the governmental and public attention to nonprofit organizations' governance, it is not surprising that boards are offering healthcare CEOs contract terms that are demonstrably justifiable and in line with a measured fair market value.

Financial Challenges

Each year, ACHE surveys members who are hospital CEOs regarding the most pressing issues facing their organizations. In 2008, as in the two previous years, financial challenges ranked as the top concern, far exceeding all the other issues (ACHE 2008e). The second most frequently mentioned issue, care for the uninsured, was also related to financial performance, while physician–hospital relations ranked third. Frank D. Byrne, MD, FACHE, president of St. Mary's Hospital in Madison, Wisconsin, explained why this combination of challenges is particularly daunting. "'Really, these three concerns are all related and they're just further evidence that the shelf life of the nation's healthcare financing is reaching its expiration date. The current method of healthcare financing has been stretched to its limit and beyond'" (Evans 2008b).

Within the three top issues, respondents named specific concerns that are facing their hospitals. These specific issues underscore the risk a hospital CEO must confront to be effective. For example, "financial challenges" includes underpayment for Medicare and Medicaid patients, bad debt, increasing costs for staff and supplies, and inadequate funding for capital improvements. "Care for the uninsured" includes similar issues and adds advocating for funding as another challenge. "Physician–hospital relations" presents such challenges as competition with physician-owned facilities and physician requests for payment for service to the hospital.

Healthcare organizations are not immune from the general state of the economy. *Modern Healthcare* reporter Cinda Becker (2008, 6) noted that the economic downturn of 2008, including the collapse of the housing sector due to subprime loans, the rapid increase in the cost of energy, and the resulting credit crunch, is "at least challenging the notion that hospitals are immune from economic downturns."

In an interview with Becker, Ralph Lawson, CFO of Baptist Health South Florida, noted that the economic situation was producing erratic and inexplicable volume trends among Baptist facilities, and that in the prior year Baptist had seen its bad debt and charity care increase by 10 percent. Compounding the distressing picture was a decline in the system's investment portfolio of 10 percent, which led him to repudiate the notion that healthcare is recession proof. According to Lawson, "Volumes decline, charity care and bad debt go up and government tax receipts go down. We anticipate there will be pressure to reduce payments to hospitals from federal and state-sponsored programs" (Becker 2008, 6).

The reality of reduced payments from government sources became evident on July 1, 2008, when the state of California instituted a 10 percent provider rate cut only six months after Governor Arnold Schwarzenegger had proposed a comprehensive healthcare reform plan (Vesely 2008a).

These ominous financial signs may herald especially challenging times for independent hospitals. Since 2000, there have been only two years in which the number of hospital bond ratings that were upgraded surpassed the number of bonds that were downgraded. In 2007, there were 26 issues downgraded and only 17 upgraded. Bond issues of healthcare systems are disproportionately highly rated, compared with those of stand-alone hospitals. In 2007, 60 percent of system bond issues rated AA+, AA, AA−, or A+, while only 19 percent of independent hospitals enjoyed such ratings. More costly access to capital also can hurt an organization's market position and future viability if it is unable to upgrade an aging physical plant, recruit physicians, or fund desired programs and facilities (Arrick 2008). Thus, CEOs of stand-alone hospitals may face greater financing and operating risks than their counterparts in system hospitals and may be more insistent on having the benefits an employment contract can afford them and the organization.

The next chapter considers the organizational and individual benefits of executive employment contracts.

CHAPTER 2

Benefits of Executive Employment Contracts

EXECUTIVE EMPLOYMENT CONTRACTS can benefit healthcare organizations and the executives they employ. In 1986, ACHE interviewed more than a dozen CEOs, consulting experts, and trustees about executive employment contracts. The study was designed to provide a balanced view of what a contract can and cannot accomplish from the perspectives of the healthcare organization and the executive.

In 2000, ACHE again interviewed executives and consultants in executive search, outplacement, and executive compensation. The results, combined with findings from a review of healthcare and general management literature, reaffirmed the individual and organizational rationale for entering into executive employment contracts. In 2008, ACHE surveyed hospital CEOs regarding their perceptions of the nature and benefits of executive employment contracts. The results of that survey are presented in Appendix A.

Leading a healthcare organization is difficult and fraught with risk. Attracting and retaining an effective executive benefits the organization, as does a clear process for executive transition. The organization also benefits from having an executive who is empowered to take risks and to lead the organization through needed changes that may cause short-term loss of support.

THE ORGANIZATION'S PERSPECTIVE ON THE BENEFITS OF CONTRACTS

As employment contracts for CEOs and other senior executives became more common throughout the 1990s, boards and executives became more sophisticated in their use (Dye 2001). As a result. contracts were designed to protect the executive and the organization. Earlier agreements had tended to favor the executive. From an organizational perspective, the following four interrelated areas are often improved in the presence of an executive employment contract (Weil and Mulholland 1989; Schaefer 1989):

1. executive decision making
2. governance
3. environmental adaptation
4. symbolic value

Each of these four benefits is discussed below.

1. Improved Executive Decision Making

Leading a successful healthcare organization is challenging and involves risk. Changing external demands and mounting internal pressures call for leaders who confidently assume prudent risks, embrace opportunities involving significant change, and lead with decisiveness. Contractual protections allow the executive to pursue decisions that are closely related to the organization's mission and strategic goals with less concern for short-term consequences of unpopular decisions.

A CEO with a contract can exert stronger leadership with the board and the medical staff, since the contract relieves the concern that a decision might result in loss of earnings. A contract with sufficient severance provisions can reduce the personal financial consequences of suddenly losing the position. This can foster an innovative management style—the type of leadership that is essential for a troubled organization and desirable for all organizations in times of rapid change.

A contract gives an executive more freedom to implement innovations, such as new products and services that enhance community well-being or improvements that contribute to the organization's viability. Researchers note that, facing an increasingly competitive, capital- and human resource–constrained environment, "those organizations that are prepared to innovate are the ones that will retain the support of the community and attract the financial resources needed to ensure success" (Weil and Mulholland 1989, 73).

A hospital chief executive related his experience in the following account (Notebaert 1986):

> I think that probably the most important thing for an executive contemplating a change in employment, or looking at the challenges in his present employment, is the issue of how to protect against the huge risks associated with the executive doing his job properly. And having that protection will help remove the barriers that discourage an executive from turning in a proper performance for his employer, which may consist of things that are not in the best interests of the chief executive. This is particularly true as we look at the changes going on around us. I think there is a need for something to protect the executive from economic harm, in the event the executive goes ahead with the right things for the hospital, which may result in his own demise. You can call that a contract if you will, but it's a focus on what will happen to protect the executive if something goes wrong. On the positive side for the hospital, you ensure that you get the very best from your executives by providing economic protection for them.

Finally, executives with employment contracts can be more objective when the hospital is contemplating a change in organizational control and ownership. A CEO with contractually guaranteed separation payments in the event of a merger, consolidation, or affiliation can evaluate such a proposal with much less bias (and be less likely to work against it) than someone who has no provision for financial well-being. Contracts may not entirely eliminate personal considerations, but they certainly can minimize them.

2. Improved Governance and Leadership Continuity

A contract can clearly set forth the employment relationship between the board and the CEO, as well as the duties and responsibilities of each. As a result, the board can focus on its fiduciary responsibilities: serving the community, ensuring quality, promoting long-term financial health, and safeguarding corporate assets. When a board recognizes and respects the CEO's responsibility for all aspects of operations, the quality of governance leadership improves. As AHA's Center for Healthcare Governance reported in its 2008 monograph of best practices for effective CEO–board relationships, "Once again, both the CEOs and the chairs stressed the importance of the board recognizing its responsibility to focus on policy and strategy and not to delve into operations" (Cohen 2008, 11).

A chairman of a health system board made the following observation on the mutual benefit to the executive and the board of a contract (Steiger 1994):

> I think that the contract is an incentive for an outstanding performance and certainly that's one of the benefits of having a contract. Secondly, I feel that contracts give you a continuity of management for a known period of time so that you can proceed and do your planning and do the administrative things that you have wanted to accomplish. You are not living with any uncertainty, either from your executive's or your board's perspective. They can put that kind of concern aside and do the work that has to be done.

A 2004 study of the effects of hospital CEO turnover demonstrates the cost of losing leadership continuity. The survey revealed several ways that a change in executive leadership can be disruptive. These included (1) competitors taking advantage of the situation by recruiting away key employees and physicians; (2) a potential delay or complete halt in important activities, such as community outreach, physician recruitment, strategic planning, and new service development; and (3) other key executives departing, including associate or assistant administrators/vice presidents, chief medical officers, and COOs (Khaliq, Thompson, and Walston 2006).

By helping to attract and retain talented and innovative CEOs, executive employment contracts improve a board's ability to appoint and evaluate the CEO. A contract can retain a competent and innovative CEO who might otherwise be recruited by a competing institution. A contract is particularly important in attracting a candidate from the limited pool of healthcare executives with demonstrated success in today's challenging environment.

Two noted healthcare compensation consultants have emphasized the importance of a contract in attracting talent. Donald C. Wegmiller, FACHE (2001b), chairman emeritus of Integrated Healthcare Strategies, commented,

> In today's health care environment, I think both boards and CEOs understand the need for employment agreements more than ever. Both parties want to be certain they have communicated their agreements accurately, and one of the best ways is to develop a well-written employment agreement. Surely, the ability of the board to attract a talented CEO will be increased with the development of an employment agreement.

Tim Cotter (2001), a healthcare compensation consultant for over 32 years, was even more emphatic:

> In my experience, boards of more sophisticated healthcare organizations expect to provide a contract to any newly hired CEO. Given

the current environment and contemporary compensation practice, they would be unlikely to attract an experienced, well-qualified candidate without such an agreement. However, severance provisions may be less generous going forward.

The use of an employment contract will help align the organization's recruitment and retention policies with industry policies. In the current health administration climate, executives are often held to the same standards of performance as chief executives in industry. In an organization whose survival is threatened, a highly competent CEO will seek the firm support of the board in the form of a contract. Many highly qualified candidates will shun jobs without such backing.

Still another advantage for the board is related to its responsibility to evaluate the CEO. An employment contract can clarify performance requirements and the evaluation process to ensure that executives are fairly judged (ACHE and AHA 1993).

3. Environmental Adaptation

An executive employment contract can help the organization adapt to a changing environment. The traditional role of CEOs has undergone significant expansion; they now face new and more complex responsibilities. Executive employment contracts can empower CEOs to undertake the needed change and reasonable risks associated with leading increasingly complex organizations.

For example, the shift away from single hospital operations to a diversified and integrated network of service delivery—a more comprehensive and complex corporate structure—has expanded the role, responsibilities, and risks the CEO assumes. In its best practices study, the AHA reported that about 40 percent of a hospital CEO's time is spent dealing with conflict (Cohen 2008). Conflict can result from competing economic blocs within healthcare organizations or from disagreements with the organized medical staff. Many a CEO has felt the heat of physicians' anger after making bold decisions that benefit the organization but prove controversial within the medical community. It is generally acknowledged among CEOs that the medical staff is the last to leave after a major conflict. It is much easier to replace a CEO. The protection of a contract helps level the playing field.

Such forces as competition with physician-owned facilities and physician requests for payment for service to the hospital have increased uncertainty and made conflict over the role and functions of the medical staff more likely. Dan Ford, an executive search consultant, has strongly emphasized the growing importance of CEO–physician relations—including collaboration, partnering, affiliations, and employment—and the way the changing structure of healthcare delivery has created a greater need for doctors in management positions (Ford 2001). He notes that the changing role of physicians has put more pressure on the CEO, who is blamed for those changes. In one sense, healthcare CEOs are in the same position as major-league baseball managers—scorned when the players do not perform or are restless, and only rarely reaping praise when they are successful.

In addition, a contract can benefit an organization by requiring confidentiality of CEOs who leave. A hospital cannot allow its strategic objectives to be revealed to a neighboring healthcare facility if it is to remain an effective competitor. A contract can also contain more stringent provisions that aid organizational viability, such as covenants of noncompetition and prohibitions against a departing CEO recruiting other key employees from the organization. Intellectual property clauses covering new ideas contributed by the CEO are a new and further extension of confidentiality requirements (ACHE 2008a).

4. Symbolic Value

The fourth—and most valuable, yet least tangible—advantage that CEO contracts can bring to organizations is their symbolic value.

A contract communicates the board's expectation that the CEO will take prudent risks and make innovative decisions that allow the organization to thrive and fulfill its mission. In addition, the contract communicates to the medical staff and to others that the CEO has the strong backing of the board.

In its 2008 survey of hospital CEOs, ACHE found that 73 percent agreed or strongly agreed (with 19 percent being neutral) that one benefit of having a contract was that it increased their ability to take necessary risks. (See Appendix A.) However, not all organizations offering CEO employment contracts fully benefit from their potential symbolic value. Only 45 percent agreed or strongly agreed (with 34 percent being neutral) that a contract enabled them to exert more forceful leadership with the board or corporate office, and 42 percent agreed or strongly agreed (with 30 percent being neutral) that a contract communicates to the medical staff that the CEO has strong backing from the board or corporate office (ACHE 2008a).

Organizational Concerns

While the potential organizational benefits of executive employment contracts are significant, some healthcare organizations may be concerned that a contract will obligate payment if a CEO is terminated or that the contract may imply tenure or a guarantee of unbridled authority.

A contract should never be viewed as an instrument for granting tenure to the executive. In offering a contract, a board does not renounce the right to terminate an executive if it believes such a move is in the best interest of the organization. In fact, by offering a contract that explicitly describes an appropriate severance policy, the board reduces the organizational risks associated with termination of a CEO. The statement that a CEO can be removed "for cause" should be avoided, because it could lead to litigation. The

CEO's contract should allow the board to terminate the CEO's contract at will. Payment of severance pay serves as a brake against arbitrary termination. This will also prevent potentially expensive and embarrassing lawsuits over whether there was sufficient cause for termination.

Nothing in a contract alters the basic relationship of the CEO with the board. To the extent that a contract enhances innovation and risk taking on the part of the CEO, such initiatives are always within the context of organizational objectives and decision-making processes and the board oversees them as appropriate.

THE EXECUTIVE'S PERSPECTIVE ON THE BENEFITS OF CONTRACTS

Just as it benefits the organization, an executive employment contract can benefit the individual in the following four key areas:

1. providing a degree of financial security
2. formalizing the relationship between the CEO and the organization
3. emphasizing the CEO's role as an organizational strategist
4. motivating the board to establish a systematic performance evaluation (Weil and Mulholland 1989)

The following sections examine these positive features in detail.

1. Income Protection

Although it does not offer complete income protection, a contract can soften the blow of sudden termination, whether it is related to issues within one's own organization or market consolidation. A contract may also check any precipitous action by the board, assuming it provides for an appropriate severance process and compensation. This may be particularly important to a CEO of a nonprofit organization, who does not have stock options or bonuses to provide financial support during a job search.

In ACHE's 2008 study of hospital CEO perceptions regarding employment contracts, respondents agreed that contracts provide important protections in the face of key organizational changes. Eighty-seven percent agreed or strongly agreed that a contract provided adequate protection in the event of involuntary separation; 74 percent felt that it adequately protected them in the event of a change in control such as a merger or acquisition; and 74 percent felt that it gave them security when board or corporate office leadership changed (ACHE 2008a).

The following personal observation by a healthcare executive from New England illustrates why the financial protections of an executive employment contract are so important (Christoforo 2000).

> We've had a surprising number of affiliations throughout New England. We have had some fairly prominent examples of mergers or alliances that failed. In managed care, too, there has been some overly eager expansion that has proven ill-advised.
>
> In our own case, a solid independent community hospital, we created a community built healthcare system that would ultimately reduce the need to keep all the existing top executives from the partner hospitals. With the advantage of a contract offering some financial protection in case of a change of control, it was less difficult to accept the change and then move on to an unfamiliar leadership position in the new organization even after dedicating years to the same hospital in the same community with the same team.

The actual extent of financial protection can vary depending on the specific market and financial position of the organization. The higher the perceived risk, the more favorable the contract an executive will likely attempt to negotiate.

2. Formalizing the CEO–Employer Relationship

A contract formalizes the relationship between the CEO and the organization. Together with a formal job description and a process for developing annual objectives, an employment contract protects the executive and the organization by detailing responsibilities and accountabilities.

As Weil and Mulholland (1989, 76) noted, "Broadly stated accountabilities and specific reporting relationships serve to ensure that the CEO is aware and responsible for the effective functioning of the organization." With a contract, both parties have agreed that provisions are reasonable and unambiguous and that either party can challenge a misinterpretation of responsibilities, should difficulties arise. A contract also ensures that the executive's role requirements cannot be diluted, and it preserves the dignity of the CEO, who has assurances protecting against a "humiliation ploy," such as being told to report to a subordinate.

The head of a community blood center in a major metropolitan area expressed why these benefits are valued. His experience illustrates that a contract not only helps specify what the board expects of the CEO, but also that a CEO with a contract feels more confident that he will be treated fairly when the going gets tough (Morand 1994).

> What [an executive employment contract] has done for the orga-
> nization is to clarify expectations. . . . Boards want good things to
> happen, but they need to specify what those good things are. And
> when you put a contract together, what it says is "Here's the role.
> Here's the responsibility. Here's the relationship. Here's what we,
> the board, expect of this individual."
>
> And the individual says, "That's fine. In return, here's what
> I expect." It's all in black and white. Because questions do come
> up, particularly as the environment heats up, and competition
> increases among institutions. And, due to market forces, there are
> a lot of questions about the viability of any healthcare organiza-
> tion. Then as the emergency heats up, there comes the question

of "Hey, what are we paying her for anyway? Why is she there?" And with a contract, it's all spelled out so that it makes it more rational. Boards don't panic. They don't fly to the switch. And as a career executive, there is the clear knowledge of what I am expected to deliver. I think it is a great way to ground a relationship in a business partnership.

Unfortunately, the advantage of clarifying expectations may exist more often in theory than in fact. In AHA's 2008 best-practices study, 82 percent of CEOs said they were not given a list of performance expectations when they were hired. "CEO and board chair responses to this same question were in general agreement. In the vast majority of cases, CEOs were not given a written list outlining their performance expectations when hired. They may have been given a job description at that time along with some discussion of key issues, but these usually lacked specifics" (Cohen 2008, 12). This finding seems in accord with ACHE's survey of hospital CEOs, which found that only 50 percent of respondents agreed or strongly agreed with the statement, "my contract is very specific about what is expected of me as CEO" (ACHE 2008a).

Regardless of the specificity of an employment contract and associated documents, such as the formal job description, the contract itself does not imply tenure or job security. Even though respondents to the ACHE study of hospital CEOs overwhelmingly felt that employment contracts provided protection in the face of change, contracts were not necessarily viewed as important for actual job security, with 49 percent agreeing or strongly agreeing to the statement, "what's most important is knowing that my job is secure for the next few years" (ACHE 2008a).

3. The CEO's Role as Principal Strategist

A contract can underscore the CEO's role as the organization's principal strategist. The financial protection of a contract can strengthen a CEO's hand in decision making, decreasing the executive's vulnerability to attack and allowing him or her to make difficult choices, take prudent risks, and espouse potentially unpopular views. An executive with a contract may be more likely to tackle issues that are not only important to the organization, but also are considered highly sensitive by the medical staff, the governing board, or members of the community. Furthermore, a relatively long severance period may keep minor disagreements from being blown out of proportion.

While financial security was clearly the most significant advantage that hospital CEOs identified in the 2008 ACHE survey, a significant segment of CEOs perceive their contract as helping to establish their leadership position. Among the respondents with contracts, 73 percent agree or strongly agree that employment contracts increased their ability to take necessary risks. On the other hand, there was less agreement on specific situations. Only 49 percent of the respondents felt that a contract gave them greater freedom to implement new programs and services; 45 percent felt they could exert more forceful leadership with the board or corporate office; and 42 percent felt that the contract served to communicate to the medical staff that the CEO had the strong backing of the board or corporate office (ACHE 2008a).

4. Systematic Performance Evaluation

A contract can specify the nature of the evaluation process. A well-designed, ongoing system for measuring leadership effectiveness and the attainment of established objectives ensures that the CEO understands the board's performance expectations and receives feedback. Such a process increases communication between the board and the CEO and ultimately improves the functioning of the organization.

A 1993 book on CEO performance evaluations (ACHE and AHA 1993, 3) noted that the performance evaluation cannot be treated as a one-directional process that has no impact on hospital governance. An effective working relationship between the board and the CEO is essential to the hospital's success.

Several factors determine the success of this relationship. First, the CEO and board must share a common understanding of the hospital's mission, its strategic plan, its goals and objectives, and its programs. Second, there must be a reasonably clear assignment of the board's and the CEO's respective responsibilities. Finally, the CEO must have an employment contract. In addition, a strong, personal relationship built on trust between the board and CEO helps resolve ambiguities that may arise.

While an executive employment contract probably would not contain specific objectives, it can provide the parameters of the evaluation process. These include the establishment of annual objectives and priorities in conjunction with the job description and minimum requirements for the feedback process.

Growth in the prevalence of annual CEO evaluations has been steady. In 1983, ACHE found that 83 percent of hospital CEOs were evaluated annually, and 46 percent had preestablished written criteria. By 2006, 95 percent of hospital CEOs reported being evaluated annually and 79 percent had preestablished written criteria (ACHE 2007). Preestablished criteria, such as a timetable for expected achievements, can protect the CEO from being unfairly discharged if the institution is in a grave financial situation and a panicky board seeks instant results.

A 2008 study found that having a performance evaluation process in place does not necessarily mean it is done well or is always viewed as beneficial to the executive. The study found that compared with 95 percent of CEOs of systems belonging to a parent organization, only 66 percent of CEOs of independent systems felt that "the CEO evaluation process establishes clear performance expectations and assesses the CEO's actual performance fairly" (Prybil et al. 2008, 30). ACHE's professional policy statement on evaluating CEO performance provides basic recommendations for a board to follow in developing its CEO evaluation process (ACHE 2008b).

Executive Concerns

In ACHE's 2008 survey of hospital CEOs, the vast majority of respondents without a contract preferred to have one, with 72 percent stating that it was the board/corporate office's policy not to offer one and only 6 percent indicating that the absence of a contract was their own preference. (An additional 23 percent said it was both their own and their board/corporate office's preference.) Only 29 percent of the respondents without a contract agreed with the statement, "our severance policy gives me all the security I need" (ACHE 2008a)

Some CEOs who prefer not to have a contract argue that a contract infringes on the trust between the CEO and the board. Others contend that contracts chill the human relationships that bind an executive to an organization. They do not want these relationships reduced to a written document. However, this appears to be a minority viewpoint, with 62 percent of respondents without a contract in the 2008 ACHE survey disagreeing with the statement, "a contract would call into question the special relationship of trust that I have with my board/corporate office" (ACHE 2008a).

Some CEOs fear that a contract will restrict their mobility and their freedom to recruit former staff to join them in a new organization. However, ACHE found that 75 percent of respondents with noncompete clauses in their contracts agreed or strongly agreed with the statement, "the contract's 'non-compete' requirements are reasonable" (ACHE 2008a). The perception of reasonableness may be further enhanced by the awareness that overly broad noncompete clauses are difficult to enforce.

Additional CEO concerns may emerge if the contract becomes disproportionally focused on protecting the organization. For example, one participant in a series of focus groups held by ACHE commented that "his employment contract represented more of a list of things he could not do rather than what he was expected to do" (e.g., clauses governing participation in outside boards) (ACHE 2008a). ACHE believes that the board and the CEO should develop a balanced contract, including organizational and individual protections, with clauses addressing compensation, benefits, perquisites, professional development, participation in outside activities, confidentiality, and ethical behavior (ACHE 2008d).

Finally, Dan Ford has suggested that seeking an employment contract can have serious negative consequences for a CEO whom the board perceives as underperforming (Ford 2001). In such a case the board may carefully examine the CEO's position and decide in favor of termination. Or, Ford adds, the board may also say, "Yes, we're going to do it, but we're going to raise the level of expectations for the CEO; which, frankly, is usually the right action to take and message to send" (Ford 2001).

Just as a marginally performing CEO might not benefit from a contract, a contract should not give a CEO a false sense of job security. For example, by providing the board with an easily accessed termination procedure, contracts may actually lead to increased CEO instability (Alexander, Fennell, and Halpern 1993). An employment agreement with severance provisions does not change the situation if the board perceives the CEO as consistently failing to meet job expectations. In fact, a CEO's sense of complacency can make matters worse, a fact that is best mitigated by a well-designed performance evaluation process with ongoing feedback.

EMPLOYMENT CONTRACTS FOR OTHER KEY EXECUTIVES

According to search consultant Carson F. Dye, FACHE (2001),

Not only have we seen an increased number of CEOs with employment contracts surface in the 1990s, but we have also seen additional senior executives such as COOs and CFOs receive employment contract protections as well. . . . Three primary factors have driven the increase in the use of employment contracts—the marketplace, the increase in the number of mergers and acquisitions and the increase in the sophistication of boards and executives about the use of contracts.

In ACHE's 2008 survey, 43 percent of CEOs with a contract reported that they offered a contract to at least one other senior executive, most often the CFO (33 percent) or the COO (26 percent) (ACHE 2008a). Even though fewer than half of the CEOs who have contracts offer them to other senior executives on their teams, most CEOs—including those who do not offer them—regard such contracts positively. For example, two-thirds of all respondents with a contract agreed that offering non-CEO executives a contract can help recruit valuable talent, and 58 percent agreed that contracts can help retain non-CEO executives. SullivanCotter's 2008 survey reports that of those health systems with employment agreements, 75 percent and 72 percent include COOs and CFOs, respectively, compared with the 68 percent and 63 percent reported in its 2000 survey (Sullivan, Cotter and Associates, Inc. 2008).

As Dye points out, the trend toward contracts for senior-level managers continues because organizations often prefer formalized employment relationships. In Dye's (2001) words, "They seek not only to minimize the direct expense and ill will caused by reductions in workforce, but to limit exposure to civil suits brought by former employees claiming unjust dismissal or wrongful discharge." Another source noted that "outside of the healthcare industry, the use of employment contracts for executives is quite commonplace. These companies often use them to minimize the possible ill will and expense caused by terminations and civil suits brought by former executives claiming unjust dismissal or wrongful discharge. It is quite rare to find senior leaders within the

Fortune 500 without some form of legal employment agreement" (Nye 1988).

As with CEOs, contracts for other senior executives may serve as the basis for the performance review process. A contract also can help protect the organization from disclosure of confidential information, and a severance clause may prevent top management from being an obstacle to a needed merger, consolidation, or affiliation. However, in the 2008 ACHE study, over half (56 percent) of the respondents stated that an actual contract for non-CEOs is not needed as long as there is a clear and fair policy on severance. Ford (2001) notes that while perhaps contracts are more frequently being granted to persons below the CEO level, he believes that those executives are probably receiving severance agreements rather than actual contracts.

While only a third of the ACHE study respondents thought that contracts for their senior executives could help facilitate mergers and other consolidations, in some cases a contract is clearly beneficial. Jeffrey Wendling (1994), former president/CEO of Northern Michigan Regional Health System, relates his organization's experience with developing contracts for other senior executives while discussions for affiliation were proceeding.

> There's tremendous uncertainty for all healthcare executives. We had a somewhat unique situation here that most hospitals don't have in that we were associated with a 125-physician multispecialty group. It was a separate organization, but they represent about 85 percent of our medical staff. That is different than you would find in most hospitals, and as a result of that, there are some interesting dynamics between the two organizations. At the time I talked to the board about extending my contract for three years, as well as introducing contracts to the immediate executive team that reports to me, we were in the middle of affiliation discussions with this clinic. I said, "I don't know what the fallout's going to be. I don't know if any of us are going to have jobs when this is all done,

but you want us to negotiate in good faith so you need to give us some protection." Our board was very amenable to that.

In the words of Jack R. Schlosser, FACHE (2001), Managing Director, SpencerStuart,

> Boards should want their key executives secure in the fact that they and their families are buffered from events that threaten their livelihood in the short or near term. Having a contract with provisions that provide a safety net will help to insure that their CEO and management team concentrate on the business at hand, and not on protective and unproductive survival strategies.

Schlosser (2001) also points out the importance of contracts for recruitment given the particular risks that senior executives, such as CFOs, face during a CEO transition.

> There is increasing attention on the financial health of the organization these days as hospitals and health systems struggle to compete. CEO turnover often occurs during times of financial stress, and when the CEO leaves it is not uncommon for his or her replacement to bring in their own Chief Financial Officer. Qualified CFOs are in great demand, and to attract the best, some type of contract or agreement is often the price of admission.

Elwood Currier (1986), former administrator of Yoakum Community Hospital in Yoakum, Texas, further notes the importance of contracts for senior executives whose positions are highly sensitive to the current CEO.

> This is a smaller hospital, so the only persons I would consider for a contract would be the Director of Nursing and the Chief Financial Officer. I think that those people serve at will, and are subject to the personality of the CEO.

It would be in everybody's best interest if they were free to speak exactly what they are thinking. They might be encumbered by job security from doing what they feel is correct. We don't want the traumatic situation which will come from both parties being angry; the CEO saying, "Here I'm going to fire you without cause," and litigation [ensues] against the hospital because of an implied contract fight. You can avoid all of those things if you first recognize that this environment is very competitive: both risk-laden and pressured. Such circumstances certainly dictate that for the protection of all concerned, there be a contract negotiated.

While contracts for subordinates may parallel the CEO's contract, the top executive faces greater risks and decision-making responsibilities. The subordinate members of the top management team must be accountable to the chief executive officer alone—not to the board—and the CEO must have the authority to terminate them without board approval. Otherwise, the CEO's authority can be circumvented by subordinates who "end run" around the CEO to the board. A hospital CEO describes how he dealt with such a situation when he developed contracts for his subordinates (Thomas 1986).

We now have a contract for my Chief Financial Officer which is very similar to my own, and then we have an in-house policy that covers the amount of severance we give to different levels of executives. While they do not have a contract or letter of employment, there is this policy that covers them up to a maximum of six months severance, but termination is still at the will of the Chief Executive Officer.

I think this is a good solution, because if I open the issue of contracts much beyond my CFO, I'd get a constant hassle of how far down to go with employment agreements. By making it broad enough, I've given people a pretty good comfort level. They know that if I'm going to make the decision to terminate them, it's going to cost the hospital, and I'm certainly going to have to think it through. Plus, it has some historical precedent at this institution, so I used a historical precedent which I thought made some sense and turned it into a formalized policy.

There seems to be ample benefit to the organization in providing a contract or letter of agreement and a related severance policy to executives beyond the CEO level.

A model letter of agreement for healthcare organization senior executives is included in Appendix F.

SUMMARY

In the introduction to its Professional Policy Statement "Terms of Employment for Healthcare Executives," ACHE (2008d) notes that

> leading a successful healthcare organization has become increasingly challenging and fraught with risk. In response to changing external demands and mounting internal pressures, healthcare organizations require a senior management team whose members can confidently assume prudent risks, embrace opportunities involving significant change and lead with decisiveness. . . . Providing executive employment contracts for the chief executive officer and other key members of senior management is one tool that a governing board can use to retain and recruit capable and unwavering leadership during such an era of change and challenge.

In addition to benefiting the individual executive, executive employment contracts can benefit the organization, increasing its ability to implement change and successfully pursue its mission.

CHAPTER 3

Process and Issues in Contract Negotiations

VARIOUS PRESSURES are transforming the organization and delivery of institutional healthcare in the United States. These pressures have accelerated the trend toward employment contracts for healthcare CEOs and other executives. They have increased the risk for and vulnerability of healthcare executives who must make difficult and controversial decisions in response to environmental changes. Even decisions made in the best interests of the organization can adversely affect the economic livelihood of the executive who lacks the financial protections of an employment contract. This chapter reviews current practices, contract elements, and the delicate process of negotiating contracts.

ASKING FOR A CONTRACT

Changes in the healthcare industry have affected the burden and risk executives need to assume in their roles. Developments over the past few years have probably exacerbated this trend. In spite of the uncertain climate and the increase in contracts, opinions differ about asking for a contract.

On the positive side, Jeffrey T. Wendling (1994), former president/ CEO of Northern Michigan Regional Health System, observed,

I don't know that it's any more risky [to raise the issue]. I think boards are more aware of the need and understand the reasons why, and they are not as reluctant to explore developing contracts with their CEOs.

Similarly, J. Larry Tyler, FACHE (2002, 126), an executive recruiter, suggests to candidates that

as soon as you have been offered the position, you can suggest using a formal employment contract as one of your conditions of employment. Hospital boards are more familiar with them than they were in the past and, in fact, may introduce the topic as a part of the job offer if they believe that you expect it.

A lawyer, consultant, or recruiter can raise the subject of a contract to avoid giving the impression that the employee does not trust the new employer. Alternatively, a candidate can simply state that a contract helps clarify points and deal with any contradictions or important omissions in the employment arrangement.

Since board members often work under employment contracts, they should realize the importance and worth of such documents. Jack R. Schlosser (2001) believes that employment contracts are even easier to discuss in the current environment.

Volunteers are the backbone of the healthcare industry, and healthcare board volunteers include many senior business leaders. Boards expect their executives to act in a businesslike manner, and a quid pro quo in recent years includes the benefits that go with increased professionalism. Downside protection for the executives on the "front lines" has come to healthcare like so many other industries. Organizations looking to attract the top tier executives quickly recognize this.

Schlosser further notes that healthcare governing bodies, especially those of healthcare systems, have become more sophisticated, thanks in part to such organizations' concentration on board development. These boards understand the importance of insulating CEOs from environments charged by emotion and politics. Nevertheless, boards seem aware that a CEO's protection can exist only so long as the CEO's behavior conforms to appropriate ethical and legal standards. Schlosser provides this observation as evidence that boards may be moving toward contract terms that are demonstrably justifiable and not extreme (Schlosser 2008).

Tim Cotter (2001) also spoke to this point.

In my experience, the board's willingness to grant a contract to the current CEO is highly correlated with its assessment of that individual's performance and his/her long-term value to the organization. A board that values its CEO and views him/her as critical to achieving the organization's near-term objectives is more likely to view a contract as a way to reinforce its assessment and to encourage him/her to maintain commitment to the organization. If the board has questions about the CEO's performance or views it as mediocre, it is far less likely it would devote the time, money, and energy required to enter into an arrangement which will limit its discretion and potentially increase its costs in the event that the CEO is terminated.

Cotter (2008b) also notes that with the scrutiny focused on executive compensation in general and on the healthcare sector specifically, boards are increasingly reluctant to enter into arrangements that may have significant future costs if a CEO change is required.

The message, then, is that the CEO should have a good understanding of the board's opinion of him or her and of board sensitivities regarding executive compensation. A board that finds the existing CEO's work acceptable but not necessarily outstanding may decide to test the marketplace when presented with a contract demand.

Therefore, the incumbent healthcare executive has to be keenly aware of his or her individual situation and relationship with the board before asking for a contract. The particular circumstances will determine the executive's negotiation strategy. For example, some boards will be more receptive than others, and a CEO doing a superior job might find negotiating easier than one who has turned in a mediocre performance. Certainly, the latter has more to worry about than a contract.

USING LEGAL COUNSEL

It is usually advisable for a CEO to obtain legal counsel. According to *Forbes*, "Employment contract law is a tiny specialty practiced by labor, tax or 'intellectual property' attorneys" (Fisher 1984). Weil and Mulholland (1989) canvassed executives and consultants and found that lawyers, executive recruiters, and consultants were the most commonly cited third parties. They conclude, "Most agreed that CEOs should have expert legal counsel who can review the wording of the contract, they can suggest points that should be introduced, or they can suggest issues that must be clarified" (86). J. Larry Tyler (2008b) recommends that executives moving to a new state for employment engage legal counsel licensed in that jurisdiction and familiar with custom and practice related to employment contracts there.

The chief executive of a hospital in Ohio (Notebaert 1986) observed that

> the average CEO who is not a licensed attorney and does not have a good grasp of legal issues would probably be well-advised to seek the help of a competent attorney, because words are extremely important in these agreements and they're extremely important in the letters that go back and forth between the parties during the pre-employment period, the negotiation period. The art of drafting these things is sometimes beyond the average person unless they're trained in legal drafting. I would recommend to the person who isn't comfortable with legal concepts and legal writing to avail himself of legal help.

When an executive or board decides to use an attorney in the contract process, careful consideration must given to how legal counsel may best be used without impinging on the very delicate and critical relationship between the CEO and the board. It is important that negotiations take place in an atmosphere free of tension. The board and the executive should understand that a trusting relationship that they may have spent years developing should not suffer because of the use of an attorney. Having an attorney serve as a mouthpiece for the CEO—especially an attorney who takes an aggressive or adversarial position—should be avoided at all costs. The attorneys for the CEO and the board should serve as counselors rather than advocates during the negotiation process.

Jack R. Schlosser (2008) elaborates,

> In my experience, organizations get contracting right when in preliminary negotiations they involve an HR executive, a search committee representative and a compensation consultant with facilitating support from the executive search professional should a formal search be underway. This way, the terms relate to both local conditions as well as compensation practices more broadly. This enables the organization to protect both the organization's image and its tax status. After this, it is appropriate to involve attorneys in getting right the language of their intent.

Schlosser also advises CEOs to use their own attorneys in reviewing the agreement produced by the negotiations. This helps to ensure that the spirit and the details of the arrangement have been captured (Schlosser 2001).

Carson F. Dye (2001) notes a delicate balance between negotiating the contract terms and developing the written language that is legally acceptable and appropriate and truly captures the spirit and intent of the agreement. He counsels that the board should "have its attorney prepare the final language, but not have them involved as the negotiator." Likewise he advises the CEO,

Because of the great increase in the number of contracts in the past ten years, there are many models to review. The ACHE monograph is one that is perfectly acceptable and most search consultants have many samples in their files. While it may be helpful to have an attorney review the final contract, it is important that the attorney be one very experienced in this area (including not-for-profit regulations). It is also very wrong to have the attorney negotiate on behalf of you. Your new board does not want a middle person involved in this relationship.

Executives should be aware that bringing an attorney into sensitive contract negotiations may cause the board to react negatively. Donald C. Wegmiller, FACHE (2001b), advises caution based on his own experiences.

Having a third party introduced into contract negotiations usually puts both parties in an uncomfortable situation unless that individual is a trusted counselor for both the board and the CEO. The board's attorney or the attorney retained by the CEO may not fit that definition. . . . Generally, it appears more positive to not introduce attorneys into the process of negotiations until it comes time to actually draft the document. Other counselors, if necessary, can serve in an intermediary role on behalf of both the board and the CEO. Once all of the business terms and contents of the agreement have been decided and negotiations are completed, then it is an appropriate time to introduce the attorneys.

Dan Ford agrees that an attorney can be most useful during negotiations by "remaining in the background." He advises the executive to participate in negotiations with the board and to strengthen his or her relationship with the board. He added that, from time to time, an executive can "bounce" questions off his or her attorney and carry those answers and ideas back into the negotiations. "The spirit of the relationship is most important and neither party should jeopardize that. Technical details are one thing. Trust is another" (Ford 2001). Ford (2008) expands, "Trust continues to be at the heart of employment of a new CEO by the board and in discussions about and negotiations of the CEO employment agreement. This employment is the start of what all parties intend to be a strong and hopefully long term relationship."

Some executives have even used the corporate counsel to conduct negotiations. However, this should be done only with the informed consent of the CEO and the board. Jeffrey T. Wendling (1994) reports,

> Basically, we have used our corporate counsel who has done a very good job of representing my interests, as well as the hospital's. Ultimately, he's accountable, in this particular instance, to the chairman of the board, but he's done a very good job of balancing.

Alan Kopman, FACHE (1994), CEO of a medical center in New York City, reported a similar experience. "I used my corporate counsel of the hospital, and I had it reviewed by my own attorney."

It seems sensible for a CEO to have legal guidance when drafting the contract. However, to preserve trust and goodwill, the CEO should negotiate the terms directly with the board while relying on legal advice before concluding the agreement. The sensitive feelings of the board and the protection of the interests of all involved parties dictate the need for finesse and objectivity during the negotiation process.

USING EXECUTIVE RECRUITERS AND CONSULTANTS

In 1988, David Nye, a professor of management, said about industry in general,

The trend toward formal agreements, and the new uncertainties it reflects, is changing the traditional role of executive recruiters. Although they still serve the corporate client, they must help both parties realize that they must be willing to make concessions.

His comment is true of the healthcare field today.

Executive recruiters and even consultants who act as mediators between the board and the executive can be useful conduits of information about the value of contracts and their prevalence in the field. Recruiters can also clear the air of misunderstandings. In fact, one reason an organization hires an executive recruiter is to facilitate an agreement on the terms of employment, whether that includes a contract or not. A recruiter or a consultant may also be seen as less threatening and adversarial than an attorney and can usually act as an impartial go-between. Weil and Mulholland (1989, 86) observe, "Executive recruiters and consultants can facilitate an agreement between a CEO and board. Acting as 'shuttle diplomats,' these third parties can assist in the negotiating process."

Dan Ford (2008) notes,

A retained executive search consultant has a formal relationship with the hospital. . . . representing their interests. However, we can provide good ideas/counsel in the employment process because he/she has seen many such vignettes and should provide an element of fairness. That is a bias I try to bring to the table. The CEO candidate of choice always has the right to their own point of view. We can serve as good sounding boards to CEOs and counsel to the hospital board, however, facilitating a constructive information exchange, without compromising our responsibility to our client board. We can sometimes interject new ideas that the client or CEO may not have thought about, and bring a difficult situation to a very satisfactory conclusion.

Tim Cotter (2008b) adds,

In certain instances, this process may be facilitated by involving a knowledgeable third party (executive recruiter, compensation consultant, attorney) who can educate and guide the CEO and the board. This individual can provide an overview of common contractual provisions and contemporary healthcare industry practice and in the case of selected supplemental benefits with significant costs such as a supplemental retirement plan develop cost estimates for consideration by all parties. In many instances he/she can also provide market data to support intermediate sanctions compliance. In addition, he/she can help ensure that both parties fully understand each of the issues under consideration. If the third party is known and trusted by the CEO and the board, he/she is in a position to ensure that both parties receive the information they need to reach a mutually beneficial agreement that the parties can feel good about.

Cotter also notes that the compensation consultant is typically hired directly by the board or a compensation committee to comply with accepted standards of independence, so he or she serves the interests of the board.

Donald C. Wegmiller (2001a) adds,

> Many times either a board chairman or a CEO will call asking, "What is the current competitive trend on this issue?" In the process of discussion, many other elements of the negotiations can be clarified, often leading to using the neutral third party to finalize the agreement.

Consultant J. Pierce Culver III (1986) recommends using a mediating third party if (1) you don't have a recruiter, (2) your recruiter lacks experience in contract issues, or (3) a CEO does not have a contract and the board decides it is a good idea to have one.

While recognizing the usefulness of third-party mediation by recruiters or consultants, executives should keep in mind that an executive search firm is employed by the institution to operate to that organization's benefit. Health System CEO Scott C. Malaney, FACHE (2001), comments,

> In my case, the recruiter was able to act as an independent, free agent serving as a go-between with the board and me. All parties enjoyed some truly unique positive dynamics in our relationships, so in our case this arrangement worked out to the advantage of everyone.

AUTHORIZATION PROCEDURE

Seventy-six percent of the hospital CEOs who responded to ACHE's Partnership Study indicated that they were hired by the board (ACHE et al. 1993). Only 30 percent of those executives reported being evaluated by the entire board, while 44 percent were evaluated by either the board executive committee or another board committee (ACHE et al. 1993). Dan Ford (2001) asserts that it should come as no surprise that executives more often negotiate their contracts with a committee of the board, usually the executive or personnel committee. He notes that the field has moved away from one-on-one negotiations (e.g., the CEO receiving a contract over lunch with the board chairman) toward the participation of and input from other board members (Ford 2001).

According to Donald C. Wegmiller (2001b), governing boards rarely fail to delegate decision-making authority to the executive committee or compensation committee. Some committees have negotiating authority; others have authority to negotiate and to sign the agreement.

Such delegation creates new challenges, observes Dan Ford (2001).

> The CEO cannot be intimidated simply because a few more people or a committee is involved. A capable chair is wise in seeking

input from other board members, and perhaps others outside of the board. He or she should, however, be the conduit for the information and the only person exchanging information with the CEO, so communications difficulties do not arise. This may turn out to be useful to the CEO as well, in that they also have that person's best interest at heart.

Cotter (2008b) suggests that as part of the approval process in a not-for-profit organization, the organization's designated approval body for executive compensation matters should review the compensation-related terms, and it should take the necessary steps to ensure that the rebuttable presumption of reasonableness is attained.

The contract should then be filed with other essential corporate documents, such as the organization's bylaws and articles of incorporation, and a duplicate original should be given to the CEO. Legal counsel should also maintain copies. Needless to say, the terms of the contract and all subsequent amendments to it should be treated as confidentially as possible.

RENEWAL AND TYPES OF CONTRACTS: FIXED TERM, ROLLING TERM, AND INDEFINITE TERM/EVERGREEN CONTRACTS

A contract can be renewed or amended with a letter, signed by the chairperson and the CEO, stating the new terms. Negotiations for renewing the contract should begin before the contract's termination and after the executive learns that the board intends to renew it. The renewal or nonrenewal of a contract should come as no surprise if the CEO evaluation committee has met on a regular basis, has provided the CEO with feedback, and has given him or her time to take needed action. ACHE and AHA (1993, 21–22) recommend that "the [CEO's] evaluation should be a continuous, year-long process culminating in an annual performance review that contains no surprises for either the evaluators or the CEO."

Carson F. Dye suggests beginning the process at least six months before the current contract runs out and using "an outside third party (the compensation consultant generally used by the board or a trusted outside advisor) to help shepherd the process along. The key thing to avoid is the possibility of silence, which might cause the CEO to believe that looking at other job possibilities might be a wise move" (Dye 2001). This procedure should allow enough time for both parties to deal with any eventualities.

TERM OF THE CONTRACT

The length of a contract is generally specified as fixed term, rolling term, or indefinite term (or "evergreen"). With a fixed term, the contract expires on a specific date. If it is not renewed, the executive is terminated. In a rolling-term contract, the compensation, benefits, and other protection run for a specific period of time into the future (usually one to two years) with no formal termination date. A contract for an indefinite term simply continues until it is terminated.

There are also combinations of these three types. One variant is to add a rolling term to a fixed-term contract. One consultant recommended having "an initial term, for example, of three years, and then looking at it annually. That will make a lot of people uncomfortable, but in my view, it keeps the CEO appropriately on his/her toes, and I also think it's realistic for the board" (Boys 1986). Each of these options provides executives with some degree of financial security.

A potentially serious drawback to a fixed-term contract is that when the end of the term arrives, any campaign to get rid of the CEO is likely to gather momentum. With an indefinite-term contract, this is less likely.

TYPES OF EXECUTIVE EMPLOYMENT CONTRACTS

Executive contracts or agreements fall into several categories. A long-form "classical" contract includes extensive provisions for the authority and responsibilities of the executive, compensation, fringe benefits, and renewal and termination arrangements. Some experts have discerned a trend away from the overformalization of the long-form contract toward a more simplified employment agreement. For example, Jack R. Schlosser (2001) observed,

> The key to the agreement is a mutual understanding of the arrangement that both parties have agreed on. The form that this takes ranges from a simple straightforward letter of agreement to a complex contract.

Dan Ford (2001) concurred,

> I think [you need] a basic list of agreed upon perquisites, benefits, and compensation without using the contract language. Once you agree on it, that basically becomes the contract, and anything you agree to becomes binding. It may be in the form of a letter, but the more you introduce formality into the contract, the more you introduce a different dimension of the relationship. Keeping out the legalese is refreshing and, again, should be in the positive spirit of the relationship. I really believe in KISS—Keep It Simple, Stupid—kinds of processes, communications and decisions, when feasible.

A short-form contract is limited to certain specifics regarding the appointment or continued employment of an executive. Basic elements of the board–CEO relationship may be defined in collateral documents, such as bylaws, personnel policies, and other policy statements. A letter of agreement may best exemplify the short form. (An example is presented in Appendix E.)

A fixed-term contract may include any of the provisions noted above, but it is written for a specified period, usually three to five years. Provisions for early termination and for renewal of the contract may be written into the document.

An indefinite-term or evergreen contract does not specify a term of employment. In accordance with stated provisions, it is subject to termination by either party at any time. J. Larry Tyler (2008b) notes that a potential drawback to such contracts is that the parties tend to simply file away the document and then lose awareness of its important provisions.

A termination or separation agreement pertains specifically to severance compensation—the compensation and related benefits to which an executive is entitled if employment is terminated. A termination agreement may be a collateral document, the principal component of an executive contract, or part of a more comprehensive contractual arrangement. (A model separation agreement is presented in Appendix G.)

Each contract form has distinct advantages and disadvantages. Boards, executives, and legal agents for both parties need to determine what is most appropriate.

ELEMENTS OF THE EMPLOYMENT AGREEMENT

No single contract is universally applicable. However, John Tarrant (1985) breaks contracts down into six basic elements.

1. Term: how long the contract runs
2. Duties: description of the job and status
3. Compensation: salaries, bonuses, stock options, etc.
4. Benefits: life and health insurance, retirement, etc.
5. Termination: who can discontinue the contract and for what reasons
6. Severance: what is paid to the fired employee

Term of Agreement

Whether to include a fixed term in the agreement is a matter for each board and executive to decide. One study found that, of hospital CEOs with fixed-term contracts, 37 percent had terms of less than or equal to one year; 19 percent had terms of one to two years; 30 percent had terms of two to three years; 4 percent had terms of three to four years; 8 percent had terms of four to five years; and only 2 percent had terms of more than five years. The median duration of terms was 24 months (ACHE et al. 1993). According to Donald C. Wegmiller (2001b), two to three years is a typical term range in healthcare, compared with somewhat longer terms for industry. Carson F. Dye (2001) noted that CEO contracts for four- to five-year terms are not uncommon. He also commented that most contracts include an automatic renewal clause that continues to renew the contract (making it an evergreen contract) unless either party takes specific action to modify it.

Persons active in the health field hold a variety of opinions about the duration of employment agreements. Weil and Mulholland (1989, 84) note that

> if a CEO is appointed for a stated term, it should be for at least five years in view of the inertia CEOs need to overcome in health care organizations; anything less than that is too short a time to accomplish objectives set forth by the board with respect to the CEO's performance.

Dye (2001) observed, however, that "virtually all contracts provide for resignation or separation, meaning in a practical sense that the length of the contract is actually less important than the length of the severance provided. In essence, as one person stated several years ago, a 100-year contract with a 30-day termination clause means that the contract is really a 30-day contract."

Jeffrey T. Wendling (1994) discusses how his board used a short-term contract as a trial period, after which it lengthened his contract.

> When I accepted this position [CEO], I asked for a contract. Even though I had been at the institution since 1983 and served as both Vice President of Professional Services and the Senior Vice President, the board initially said, "You don't have any CEO experience. We are going to give you a six-month contract and reevaluate it." It was certainly reasonable. At the end of that period, the contract was renewed for a one-year period. Then in 1992, I asked for a three-year contract, and that's what I'm still operating under.

Others believe that more attention should be paid to managing relationships, such as with the board and medical staff, than to negotiating a long-term contract. After all, regardless of the length of the term, the CEO still needs smooth day-to-day working relationships. One of the executives we interviewed (Name withheld 1986) elaborated,

> Let us assume that I had a contract for three years and it said that I would not be fired. Well, at the end of three years they can get rid of me, or they can get rid of me in the interim as long as they buy me off. So, there might be some financial protection, but what's far more important to me, and what I really think, and emphasize most strongly, is managing the relationship. I'm not suggesting that you shouldn't put protections in there for disputes with the medical staff, etc., but I am suggesting that the focus be on managing the relationship throughout the term of the contract—not on just what happens at the very end.

One hospital CEO reported that an indefinite-term contract with annual renegotiation of compensation terms strengthened relations with the board. The discussions surrounding negotiating these terms annually improved communication (Johnson 1994).

These views do not imply that if an executive has good relationships with everyone, a contract is not needed. Most executives will confront situations that require the protections a contract affords.

Given the variety of circumstances faced by the healthcare executive, the length of the term really depends on the situation. But whatever the individual circumstance, contracts that are intended to be in effect for longer than one year should either state an explicit term (usually three to five years) or state that they will continue until terminated.

Duties

The job title, the broad responsibilities that accompany it, and the reporting relationship should be explicit in the contract or, at the very least, should be referenced and added as an appendix. It helps to have the general authority of the CEO specified in the bylaws. Duties of the position could also be linked to the accountabilities that are listed in a performance evaluation.

The assignment of responsibilities needs to be clear-cut and mutually understood. The board is the hospital's legal organ of accountability, and it is responsible for selecting a CEO, ensuring the executive's satisfactory performance, overseeing the institution's financial integrity and long-term viability, adopting a corporate mission and goals, making corporate policy, and ensuring the quality of care. The CEO is responsible for long-range planning, day-to-day management, and achievement of the organization's objectives (ACHE and AHA 1993).

ACHE (2004) delineates the criteria for evaluating hospital CEOs. A regular performance evaluation is integral to the contract process. Perhaps the most direct mechanism for ensuring CEO accountability is a formal performance evaluation by the board using preestablished standards or criteria. A 2006 ACHE survey of CEOs found that approximately 95 percent of respondents are evaluated at least once a year (ACHE 2006). This compares to 63 percent reported in 1989 (ACHE and AHA 1993). Annual CEO evaluations have increased for all types of hospital ownership. Eighty-four percent of for-profit and private, not-for-profit hospitals use preestablished criteria to formally evaluate CEO performance, but a third of public hospitals do not. Larger hospitals are more likely to employ formal performance evaluations. Perhaps this is because monitoring management activity and performance is more difficult for boards of larger hospitals, and therefore these boards need formal means of establishing clarity. Formally specified goals may also help CEOs in larger hospitals sort out the multiple strategies in which they engage (Alexander et al. 1999).

Tim Cotter (2001) observes that, in his experience, the CEO's key accountabilities are spelled out on the contract directly or by reference, and the key performance measures are reinforced in the organization's annual CEO assessment process.

> Boards are increasingly comfortable specifying the areas of accountability and the outcomes to be achieved by the CEO. Attempting to tell the CEO how to do his/her job or spend his/her time through the contract or the performance assessment process is fraught with peril.

Wegmiller (2001a) explains further why specifying how executives should spend their time is inappropriate.

> First, executive time allocation will change depending upon changes in the organization strategy. Time allocation will also change depending upon size and maturity of the CEO's staff, changing role of the CEO in the community, and a host of other factors. To attempt to spell this out in an employment agreement is inappropriate. The proper place for such a discussion is in the annual performance evaluation of the CEO and the

setting of management objectives and/or CEO objectives for the coming year.

Dye (2001) notes that an employment contract can go far in preserving the self-respect and pride of an executive.

There have been examples, particularly in some merger/acquisition situations, where executives have been asked to accept significantly lower compensation or severance arrangements or reduced responsibilities simply to try to force them out. The use of a well-developed contract can provide very appropriate protection in these situations.

The executive should ensure that his or her specific authority is explicitly delineated in the job description, along with broadly stated accountabilities and reporting relationships. However, a long list of duties and responsibilities should be avoided as it could limit the authority of the CEO to manage the institution. It could also conceivably lead those who are threatened by the CEO's proposed actions to challenge his or her authority to perform functions not included on the list.

Compensation

Contemporary healthcare executive compensation packages are complex. The well-designed contract or agreement typically specifies the initial cash compensation package (salary, incentive opportunity—annual and perhaps long-term—and signing bonus) and the process for upward adjustments. It often addresses items that relate to the initial employment period, such as moving and relocation support.

Compensation is often stated as a minimum, not a maximum. The contract should not be specific about future salary increases, which are typically subject to periodic review. Flexibility is needed because of the cost-of-living index, the institution's financial condition, market conditions, and the executive's performance. One consultant recommends keeping compensation flexible so the board can react to an executive's performance, whether it be wonderful or awful (Culver 1986).

This advice applies to recruitment and retention. Nell Minow (1999) of the Corporate Library states,

> We recognize that a board must address opportunity costs in enticing an outstanding prospect. An outstanding executive who has a highly performance-based contract will not be willing to move without a clear chance to do better. This is exactly where a board is put to the test.

Wegmiller (2001a) cautions,

> Establishing exact compensation numbers and placing them in the employment agreement requires frequent modifications to the agreement. A better process is to merely state the original compensation amount plus an indication of the Board and CEO's agreement as to how frequently the compensation should be reviewed, which is most commonly an annual event.

Increasingly, salary is pegged to the performance evaluation. The CEOs of 95 percent of nonfederal, short-term general medical/surgical hospitals receive an annual performance evaluation (ACHE et al. 1993). A 2008 study of hospital governance found that 91 percent of hospital and health system boards follow a formal process for evaluating the CEO's performance (Prybil et al. 2008). The vast majority of the CEOs participating in the study state that their financial compensation is linked directly to the results of their performance evaluation (Prybil et al. 2008).

Tim Cotter (2008b) states that the growth of healthcare incentive compensation plans (found in more than 80 percent of not-for-profit health systems, according to his firm's survey of systems participating in the 2008 SullivanCotter report on Executive

Compensation in Hospitals and Health Systems) is due to the following factors:

- Not-for-profit healthcare organizations have recognized that incentives are a far more effective way to pay an organization's executives than base salaries alone. Such programs permit compensation at the upper end of the market in years in which there is strong performance and provide middle-of-the-market compensation when performance targets are not achieved. In addition, incentive awards do not represent fixed costs.
- As healthcare organizations have seen their competitors implement such programs (in the early 1980s, fewer than 5 percent of not-for-profit healthcare organizations had executive incentive programs), they are forced to implement such programs to remain competitive.

Wegmiller, and David A. Bjork, PhD (2001), comment on other factors that have led to the growth in incentive compensation plans for healthcare executives. These include

- an increasing interest on the parts of boards and executives to put an element of executive pay at risk, with the opportunity for greater reward if predetermined objectives are met;
- the desire of boards to focus executives' efforts and attention on key strategies or objectives that are critically important to the organizations' success; and
- board members' experiences in other industries of the positive effect of incentive compensation on organizational performance.

A 2007 survey published by Integrated Healthcare Strategies discusses the prevalence of incentive plans. Use of short-term incentive compensation programs among responding healthcare organizations ranged from 90 percent in independent system hospitals to

78 percent in independent hospitals. CEOs at independent systems had a median target of 32 percent of salary and a median maximum of 45 percent of salary. CEOs at independent hospitals had a median target of 30 percent of salary and a median maximum of 38 percent of salary (Integrated Healthcare Strategies 2007).

Long-term incentive programs are less prevalent in system and independent hospitals, ranging from 23 percent for systems to 11 percent for independent hospitals. CEOs eligible for short- and long-term incentives had total incentive opportunities as high as 80 to 100 percent of salary at target or expected value. Other senior executives had total incentive opportunities as high as 50 to 60 percent of salary (Integrated Healthcare Strategies 2007).

Nonprofit institutions may, with prudence, tie executive incentive compensation to the performance of the organization. Such arrangements should be approached with extreme caution because of the potential legal, tax exemption, fiscal, and public relations ramifications. For not-for-profit executives, no portion of the organization's earnings can be directed to individuals.

Since incentive compensation is increasingly being stipulated in employment contracts, more contracts require performance evaluations with specific criteria. This arrangement facilitates ongoing feedback from the board to the executive. There is a distinction between a salary increase from a performance appraisal and incentive compensation. According to Wegmiller (2001a),

> A common approach for incentive compensation goals is to establish levels of accomplishment, such as threshold, target, and maximum. The target level accomplishment is usually tied directly to the goals that have been set in the annual plan. Threshold level recognizes that accomplishments have been made but not at the plan level, say at only 90 percent with a reduced award opportunity. A maximum level is set that provides incentive for the executives to exceed the target but within a "cap" on incentive compensation payments.

Incentive plans cannot always be funded. SullivanCotter reports that 60 percent of healthcare incentive plans require a minimum level of financial performance before any incentive awards are paid, regardless of performance on the nonfinancial measures. An emerging trend has been to eliminate the financial threshold requirement. In such situations, Cotter (2001) notes, the incentive amounts are typically reduced.

Some boards use a pass/fail system for incentive compensation—an executive either makes it or does not. Other boards might tie incentive compensation to accomplishing a proportion (such as two-thirds) of objectives (Boys 1986). Incentive programs have become more defined, with limits being set. Such incentive payments are decided when signing the contract or when establishing annual performance objectives. It is better not to tie incentive compensation objectives to financial performance alone. Increasingly, such objectives are linked to a balanced set of measures. One study found that nonprofit healthcare organizations regularly tie CEO performance expectations to financial performance, patient quality and safety, leadership team building, and community benefit (Prybil et al. 2008).

Tim Cotter (2001) notes an emergence of long-term incentive plans in the healthcare sector. While still a minority practice, such programs provide incentive payments for performance over a three- to five-year period.

According to Cotter (2001), employer-provided deferred compensation is commonly included in healthcare executive compensation packages. While often viewed as only of interest to executives approaching retirement, such plans are increasingly considered an important compensation device for executives of all ages. Such programs are designed to

- improve the organization's ability to recruit executive talent;
- provide mid-career executive hires with full-service or near full-service retirement income benefits;

- make up for benefits lost due to restrictions created by Section 415 and Section 401(a) (17) limits of the IRS code;
- prevent competition by executives after termination; and
- encourage executives to stay with an organization.

The traditional tax-sheltered annuity has been available for years in tax-exempt charitable organizations. However, changes in the tax laws have reduced the amount of taxes that can be deferred by this method, so hospitals and executives have begun to employ new types of deferred compensation. One deferred compensation strategy that has gained favor in the last few years is the so-called supplemental employee retirement program, or SERP.

Unlike a qualified plan pension benefit, a SERP is (and must be, to achieve the tax deferral on the benefits associated with it) subject to a substantial risk of forfeiture. However, if properly structured, it can serve as a retention incentive and provide for the tax-deferred accumulation of funds while the executive is employed. Benefits are not taxed until the executive vests, often after a specified period of service (e.g., 5 or 10 years). According to Cotter (2009), current IRS regulations (IRC 457(f)) define the rules for setting vesting dates for deferred-compensation plans. These regulations increase the likelihood that the executive may forfeit deferred amounts (e.g., upon voluntary termination prior to vesting) and are one reason for the trend toward shorter vesting periods. If IRS-proposed regulations (issued August 2007 as IRS Notice 2007-62) are implemented, certain tax-deferral strategies (e.g., noncompete arrangements) may no longer be permitted (Cotter 2009).

So-called split-dollar insurance policies accomplish similar objectives. Industry has used such policies for decades, and they are becoming more common in healthcare executive compensation. Split-dollar policies are a form of life insurance in which two parties "split" the proceeds. Most commonly, the organization's interest in the policy is equal to the amount in premiums it has paid on behalf of the executive. The executive's interest is equal to the cash surrender value of the policy. To achieve tax deferral of the cash-surrender-value buildup, the policy is usually attached to an economic noncompete agreement between the organization and the executive (Wegmiller 2001a).

Retention incentives appeal to some hospitals, especially those with younger CEOs they wish to retain (Integrated Healthcare Strategies 2007). These incentives may provide for the payment of a lump sum if the CEO stays for a minimum period, usually no more than five years. Hospitals and their executives should exercise caution in these areas, however, due to potentially devastating tax consequences if these arrangements are improperly structured. These agreements should be put in place by competent benefits and legal consultants and reviewed by the hospital's outside audit firm before implementation.

Another popular form of compensation is a one-time sign-on bonus for the new executive tailored to the individual's needs. A sign-on bonus is especially attractive during times of economic duress. Each executive comes with financial needs that may not be fully addressed by the organization's normal compensation and benefits programs. At the senior executive level, organizations can be creative and flexible in meeting these needs. Since many executives have short-term and long-term incentive plans, a sign-on bonus can be used to make up the loss for an executive who is leaving a position in the midst of a qualifying period for an incentive payment. Similarly, an executive moving from the investor-owned sector may lose unvested options. A sign-on bonus can help offset this. An organization using a sign-on bonus is more likely to attract the executive in the time frame desired, and the executive does not need to "leave money on the table." The beauty of the sign-on bonus is its variety of uses, including supplemental dollars for moving, temporary housing, real estate issues, and guaranteed bonuses (Cotter 2001). Tyler (2008a) reports that they are often used to solve internal equity problems when the existing salary range is not adequate to attract the ideal CEO. The signing bonus allows the organization to temporarily fix the issue until internal salaries are changed or reviewed.

Dan Mulholland, an attorney who specializes in employment contracts, explains that when using sign-on assistance, it helps to be as specific as possible in describing what is and is not covered. For instance, if a "bridge loan" is being contemplated to help the recruit buy a new home while his or her old one is still on the market, the exact terms of that loan should be described. Likewise, if closing costs on the new residence or moving expenses are going to be covered, it makes sense to list them along with an estimate of how much will be spent on each item or an overall cap on how much will be reimbursed. This will avoid misunderstandings and minimize the risk that the IRS will question the "reasonableness" of the arrangement (Mulholland 1994).

Given the IRS Intermediate Sanctions regulations and public interest in and media scrutiny of executive compensation, most healthcare boards are keeping close tabs on changes in executive compensation packages. Tim Cotter (2001) notes that since board members who knowingly participate in an excess benefit transaction face personal financial penalties under Intermediate Sanctions regulations, they need to be comfortable that the compensation being paid to their key executives falls within the bounds of contemporary market practice and that the approval body takes the necessary steps to show the rebuttable presumption of reasonableness. With the new Form 990's requirement for enhanced disclosure of executive compensation practices beginning in 2008, discomfort with compensation components, such as loans and club memberships, is likely to increase.

When assessing executive compensation, it is best practice for boards or their relevant committees to review

- competitive total compensation data for comparable positions at organizations (both healthcare and nonhealthcare) of comparable size, scope, and complexity and
- publicly available executive compensation data, such as that reported on IRS Form 990.

Cotter (2001) concludes,

> Boards are facing increasingly complicated situations regarding CEO compensation. First, what kind of compensation package is necessary to attract/retain the right individual? Second, does this compensation package fall within the bounds of contemporary market practice and is it defensible on this basis? Third, what will our key stakeholders (physicians, staff, and the community) think about this package? Finally, is the institution receiving the appropriate return on the CEO compensation expenditures it has made?

These issues will certainly play a greater role in future performance evaluations and executive employment contracts.

Benefits

Contracts may specify fringe benefits and perquisites associated with the position. These benefits are often presented in separate letters of agreement between the board and the executive. Benefits are receiving more attention as competition for well-qualified candidates intensifies. Boards realize that to attract and retain the best and brightest, they need to offer packages that will stand up to the test of the marketplace (Schlosser 2001).

Table 3.1 compares the prevailing benefits and perquisites CEOs received in 2000 and 2008. Cotter (2008a) notes that with the increasing scrutiny of executive compensation and the disclosure requirements of the new Form 990, many boards are having second thoughts about benefits and perquisites that draw public scrutiny, such as club memberships, financial planning and loans, and spouse travel.

Wegmiller (2001a) observes that organizations are recognizing that their executives' personal situations vary widely. Therefore, more boards are using flexible benefit plans, which provides executives

Table 3.1 Health System CEOs' Benefits and Perquisites, 2000 and 2007

Benefit	2000	2007
Automobile	91%	81%
Car/cellular telephone	71%	50%
Country club	64%	37%
Social/luncheon club	31%	21%
Financial planning	43%	29%
Legal services	13%	14%
Supplemental life insurance	78%	82%
Supplemental long-term disability	72%	76%

with benefits options from which they can choose. In these flex plans, boards establish a percentage of base salary that is available for executive benefits. The median benefit expenditure (with paid time off [PTO]) in healthcare in 2008 was approximately 41 percent of base salary (Schoenberger 2009). Costs for basic employee benefits and any designated executive-level benefits are deducted from this total amount. What remains is used to pay for the executive's selections from a menu of individual benefit choices. Common choices include an individual professional disability insurance contract; supplemental life insurance, usually of a cash-accumulating type; spouse life insurance; long-term-care insurance; and an opportunity for a capital accumulation account. Each year, the individual executive gets to make new choices from that year's benefit allowance.

This flexible approach to executive benefit planning has several advantages.

- The board is ensured a fixed benefit cost established as part of its executive compensation philosophy.
- Individual executives can tailor their own benefit plans according to their own needs and wishes.
- Changes can be made to the benefit plans by adding benefits at any level while keeping cost within the cap established by the board.

- As an individual executive's lifestyle changes, individual benefit choices can be changed without disrupting the benefit plans for other executives or increasing costs to the organization (Wegmiller 2001a).

In granting a CEO extensive benefits, a board should avoid situations in which disclosure of contract terms would produce a public relations disaster, recognizing that some benefits will have to be disclosed on the IRS Form 990.

Matching benefits to the needs and desires of executives is an ongoing trend. Wegmiller (2001a) notes that many organizations have shifted their time-off plans to a comprehensive PTO plan incorporating vacation, holidays, sick leave, and other provisions for paid time off. This provides the executive—and all employees—with more flexibility in dealing with personal situations. Cotter (2001) reports that key benefit trends for healthcare CEOs are more generous vacation and paid-time-off allotments and enhanced supplemental life, disability, and retirement benefits. While there has been considerable talk of sabbatical leaves, few systems make them available to their CEOs. Perquisites such as club memberships are declining in popularity (Cotter 2001).

Relocation packages are standard arrangements for new executives. However, benefits such as financial assistance with real estate costs, housing arrangements, and mortgage subsidies are less prevalent than in previous years, with the exception of locations with high housing costs, such as New York City and San Francisco. However, with the current decline in real estate values, many executives are requesting signing bonuses.

Attention to the working spouse's situation is increasing. Many organizations are actively involved in providing job search and other related assistance to the spouse (Wegmiller 2001a).

Social entertainment is another controversial benefit. Business meals are more focused on business and are less frequently "old-boy" club arrangements. Some believe that personal relationships are more important today in consummating business deals. This might mean more social entertainment in the home and in the club. An opposing school of thought views club memberships as unnecessary frivolities. Judges and bureaucrats who question hospital tax exemptions are less sanguine about the need for club benefits. The SullivanCotter survey reports that 39 percent of health system executives receive country club memberships, and 23 percent receive lunch club memberships (Sullivan, Cotter and Associates, Inc. 2008). Integrated Healthcare Strategies (2007) reported 43 percent and 19 percent, respectively.

An important additional benefit is executive outplacement, received by approximately 70 percent of the CEOs in the 2008 SullivanCotter survey. One hospital CEO (Malaney 2001) comments on the importance of such a benefit:

> I feel strongly that executive outplacement is a very important benefit. In fact I would not sign a contract without it. I have been through outplacement so I know how helpful it is.

John Challenger (2008), CEO of Challenger, Gray, and Christmas, expands on the significance of this benefit.

> Because of the intense competition, and for many, the relative difficulty in finding a comparable position, executive outplacement assistance has become an increasingly popular benefit with advantages for the executive and the employing organization.
>
> Quality outplacement service is an essential element of an executive's severance package. Too many discharged executives delay or passively conduct (e.g., by looking for the perfect job) their searches until the severance is about to run out. Outplacement prevents such career-damaging behavior, creates goodwill, and averts lawsuits.
>
> Outplacement should include expert resume writing assistance, constructive career assessment, thorough interview preparation and de-briefing, and administrative support. The experienced outplacement counselor will proactively reach out to the individual on a daily/weekly basis and provide situational support and motivation.

Shortening job search times and improving the quality of the jobs found is a win-win for the discharged individual and the company.

Additionally, from the employers' side of the aisle, not only does the displaced employee gain the benefit of swifter re-employment, the organization can save money on reduced severance and benefits payments. The savings on coverage for terminated employees quickly becomes substantial.

Investor-owned companies use various equity elements to attract and retain executives, such as stock options, restricted stock grants, and stock appreciation rights. Equity participation is not possible in not-for-profit organizations. However, healthcare organizations have become creative in developing deferred-compensation plans, capital accumulation plans, retention incentive plans, and other compensation devices to attract and retain the talent they need (Wegmiller 2001a).

The most important factor for an executive to consider is how benefits really match his or her needs. Some benefits may be considered taxable income, especially when they are not available to other employees. Executives should check with their accountants or attorneys regarding personal income tax implications of fringe benefits.

Termination Situations and Provisions

The termination arrangements are the centerpiece of the executive employment contract. Terminations typically address four scenarios.

1. In the case of death, salary may continue for a specified period.
2. In the event of disability, compensation may continue in excess of the employee benefit package.
3. Termination without cause may take place if executives disagree with the board over the hospital's goals. In such

cases, no misconduct is implied, but salary usually continues for one to three years. This type of termination is probably one of the major reasons for an executive employment contract. Weil and Mulholland (1989, 82) note,

> The board must have the clear authority by contract to terminate the CEO if it desires. But if it exercises that right of termination, the agreed upon termination payments should be made regardless of the reason for termination. The danger of arbitrary termination for political or personal reasons, which was the basis for recommending termination clauses in the first place, is still real in the hospital field—perhaps more than ever in today's volatile environment. Therefore, it is probably in the best interest of the corporation, from the standpoint of assuring decisive leadership, that the termination clause be operative in all but the most egregious situations. This is not unfairly weighted in favor of the CEO, as some have suggested, rather it is in the interest of good institutional management and, thus, should be the goal of any conscientious governing body.

4. Termination with cause is restricted to serious misconduct, not just poor performance. This type of termination arrangement, the so-called for-cause or competency clause, can lead to endless litigation if not handled properly. A growing body of law challenges the traditional rule that an employee can be discharged at will without a written agreement to that effect. Hence, except for intentional illegal conduct, competency clauses are likely to pose serious problems of definition. Agreement on a definition of cause is a major drawback in competency clauses and can lead to serious problems during negotiations and during implementation of the contract. If handled less than expertly, negotiation discussions regarding the cause

of termination can quickly disintegrate, and the parties can find themselves in opposite corners wondering why their contract is not working.

Dye (2001) comments on the ineffectiveness of typical competency clauses.

One of the best reasons for the use of an employment contract is to minimize litigation—and perhaps more importantly, minimize the possibility that a dispute between the board and the terminated CEO be publicly aired. If the board wishes to terminate the CEO, that is their prerogative. And the existence of a severance agreement—a clause that requires that the board pay the terminated CEO two years of salary and benefits—may serve to better ensure that the termination decision be made logically and appropriately. A clause that attempts to define competency will often fail because there can always be an argument about competency.

He adds,

It has always been very difficult to define just cause. Is just cause a good cause, and if it is a good cause, good for whom? And how is this really determined? To define it in the depth needed to avoid litigation may necessitate much too many pages for the comfort of the typical board. It is my recommendation that, in the event of a termination, the focus be on reaching a settlement quickly rather than trying to work though the due process of determining cause.

In its original 1982 publication on contracts, ACHE made an observation that still holds true today: "Except for a provision pertaining to intentional illegal conduct, competency clauses in a termination agreement pose problems of definitions and tend to dilute the basic purpose of the agreement" (ACHA 1982). A contract should set out the rights and obligations of the executive and the organization and make explicit the conditions under which the CEO can be discharged.

However, Cotter (2008b) notes that with increasing scrutiny on executive compensation and on boards that provide significant severance payments in cases of very poor performance, CEOs should expect attempts to include properly balanced competency clauses.

In voluntary termination by the executive, all compensation and benefits stop. As a result of the Thirteenth Amendment to the U.S. Constitution, which outlawed slavery and involuntary servitude, no one can be compelled to be employed by another against his or her will, so executives can quit at any time. However, the contract can create financial disincentives or penalties for executives who quit without giving adequate notice or incentives for those who do give notice.

Change of Control and Termination

Change of control provisions deal with situations in which the organization's ownership and control is transferred to another organization, which can result in termination of key executives. This is common in mergers and needs to be addressed in the employment agreement or in a distinct separation agreement (such as the example in Appendix G).

The change-of-ownership clause should define what constitutes a change of control and the rights of the executive in such situations. Typically, there is a choice between "single-trigger" and "double-trigger" provision of termination benefits. In the single trigger approach, benefits are provided when control changes even if employment is not terminated. The double trigger requires a change of control and a termination before benefits are provided. The termination may be documented, or it may be inferred from the employer's actions—referred to as a "constructive termination" in the parlance of contract law.

According to Wegmiller (2001a):

With the rapid acceleration of mergers, affiliations, and other forms of change of control, this provision must be included in the termination section of any modern-day employment agreement. It provides both the board and the executive with definition and direction for an event that may occur a number of years in the future when boards have changed and the entire industry has changed.

Cotter (2008b) comments,

Given the experience that the healthcare industry has had with "change in control" situations, it is almost certain that the CEO will request enhanced severance protection if such an event is imminent. This makes sense for both parties, given the increased risk faced by the CEO and the board's interest in insuring that the CEO aggressively pursues all such opportunities with the organization's best interests in mind.

Apart from clauses covering the various events that may lead to termination, termination arrangements can include other clauses. Probably the best known are the so-called restrictive covenants. One kind of restriction is the noncompete or geographic clause, which forbids an executive from working at a competing facility in the area for a certain period following resignation or termination. This clause should not impose undue hardship on the employee, such as forcing him or her to either stay at the hospital or leave the area. If possible, the restriction should not last longer than the severance period. Executive recruiter J. Larry Tyler (1994) recommends that the restrictive covenant be reasonable in terms of distance, duration, and terms of work. Other experts suggested that "a restriction against a CEO taking a similar position in the hospital's service area for up to two years should be upheld" (Weil and Mulholland 1989). Restrictive covenants are unenforceable in some states.

Wegmiller (2001a) observes that noncompete agreements are a quid pro quo for the severance benefits provided in executive employment agreements. In addition, an economic noncompete agreement may provide the basis for tax deferral of some executive benefit plans. When properly defined, such agreements are reasonable protections for the organization and do not provide unreasonable restraints on an executive from seeking another position (Wegmiller 2001a).

Questioning the legal aspects of restrictive covenants and whether they would really hold an executive in his or her position, Ford (2001) asserts,

> Probably the best value they have is an "implied threat." If that is really the reason for a restrictive covenant, possibly some consideration should be given as to how conducive the use of a covenant is to a good relationship between the executive and the board. Again, what is most important is the spirit of the relationship. I believe in win-win, even in the dissolution of relationships. Beyond the breaching of confidential information, there is really nothing to be gained from threatening or attempting to prevent a person from making a living. If a board is threatened because their CEO goes across town, then the board should be challenged to go out and find a CEO even better than the one they could not keep. And, they should look inside of their own organization, and discover and evaluate what the barriers were to that departed CEO's continued successful tenure in and leadership of their organization.

Other types of restrictive covenants include confidentiality provisions that can prevent a terminated executive from taking or divulging confidential information about an institution's operation. This merely restates common law. Still other provisions may prohibit raiding key employees.

Some termination arrangements contain an arbitration requirement also known as "alternative forum for dispute resolution." This requirement allows for informal arbitration of disputed issues between the executive and the organization. The American Arbitration Association, United States Arbitration and Mediation, and the American Health Lawyers Association, among others, can provide arbitrators or mediators for resolution of disputes. This is less costly than court-mandated enforcement of the contract, but experts caution that "arbitrators often have the tendency to 'split the difference' when deciding a case, which can work to the disadvantage of a party who has a clear-cut right to relief" (Weil and Mulholland 1989, 83). Mediation, on the other hand, helps the parties resolve their dispute themselves, rather than having a solution imposed on them.

Finally, other termination arrangements require the executive who voluntarily terminates to remain on the job for some period to ensure continuity of management. Since a person cannot be forced to remain in a job, such a requirement might be enforced by causing the executive to forfeit his or her termination pay or incur some other financial penalty.

Severance

The financial arrangements negotiated in the severance clause provide economic protection to the executive so he or she can act without undue caution. Weil and Mulholland (1989, 82) note this benefit of the severance clause.

> In the interest of the board, the hospital, and the patients, the CEO must be able to exercise authority to the fullest extent possible. The CEO must also be able to make hard decisions without fear that his or her job may be in jeopardy simply because someone on the board or the medical staff dislikes the decisions for reasons unrelated to the best interests of the hospital.

Sullivan, Cotter, and Associates, Inc.'s *2008 Survey of Manager and Executive Compensation in Hospitals and Health Systems* reports that 76 percent of health systems and 61 percent of hospitals have formal severance policies for executives. Actual severance prevalence for healthcare CEOs is likely higher due to its inclusion in individual arrangements and contracts (Cotter 2001).

The Sullivan Cotter survey data indicate that severance for the CEO is a common practice, that it is typically based on salary, and that in most cases it is provided without offsets for new employment. For the CEO, the severance period typically covers 24 months, with the middle range covering 12 to 24 months. Benefits continuation typically includes health and life insurance, although the continuation of other benefits is not uncommon. To receive severance, the CEO typically has to sign a release of all claims (Cotter 2001).

The severance clause indicates the amount to be paid to the employee in the event that the board votes in favor of termination. Even though he or she is no longer working for the organization, the executive is entitled to a stated amount of salary and benefits. Probably the most important aspect of the severance clause is the amount of compensation and the period over which it will be paid.

The number of months of severance to which an executive is entitled is subject to negotiation. The amount of compensation should reflect the risk and challenges of the position and the possible difficulty of finding a comparable position. It should be sufficient to provide a counterweight to arbitrary termination. Maximum protection is afforded to the executive in a rolling contract, which provides compensation and benefits for a specified period.

Regarding the length of severance, "typically the provision is for one or two years among not-for-profit organizations and slightly longer in for-profit settings" (Schaeffer 1989, 147). In a 2005 report on severance and separation benefits covering 16 industry groups, Lee Hecht Harrison (2005) found that the hospital and healthcare services group ranked sixth in terms of generosity of separation benefits. The report also notes that unlike other employee levels, C-suite severance is generally not determined by years of service but is more commonly based on an employment agreement or negotiated on an individual basis. ACHE (2008d) recommends that severance compensation for CEOs should be paid for a minimum of 12 months, with continuation of compensation up to another six months, if needed, to find another comparable position.

Reporters for business publications have written that severance pay is coming down. Perri Capell of the *Wall Street Journal* noted that "shareholder pressure on this issue is an irresistible force that companies are going to have to respond to" (Capell 2008). Cotter (2008b) agrees that in the for-profit sector, there is a movement toward more conservative severance provisions for CEOs, and in his experience this trend is beginning to emerge in the healthcare industry.

Some organizations have begun to provide severance as a bridge to other employment. In other words, severance is not paid as a lump sum but is continued either until the terminated executive finds other employment or the period of severance expires. Often, payments will be reduced but not totally cut off if the new job pays less than the old one—making up the difference, so to speak. The practice seems, in part, to be a reaction against negative perceptions of perceived excesses of some "golden-parachute" contracts.

With the addition of noncompete and nonsolicitation clauses and mitigation for new employment tied to termination severance benefits, lump-sum payments of severance are less common. With a lump-sum payment, it is more difficult for an organization to recover payments if the executive violates such terms, and legal action is typically required.

Cotter (2009) notes that the proposed IRS regulation (issued August 2007 as IRS Notice 2007-62), if implemented, may treat all or part of severance benefits as immediately taxable, resulting in more organizations paying severance as a lump sum.

Offsets to severance benefits for earnings from other employment during the severance period are part of some employment agreements. There is no consistent pattern, and offsets are largely a matter of individual negotiation. However, it is rare to see an offset of more than 50 percent, meaning that earnings in the last half of the severance period are offset against the severance benefits (Wegmiller 2001a).

Cotter (2001) notes that while bridging provisions are not the majority practice, they are quite common. Boards are concerned about the image of paying significant severance to an individual who quickly finds a new job. As a compromise, some contracts require payment of minimum severance (12 months) regardless of the time it takes the CEO to find new employment.

In determining the content of the severance clause, the executive should make a realistic estimate of his or her most pressing needs if terminated. These needs, in turn, could be included in the negotiation process.

SUMMARY

The process of negotiating an employment contract involves a careful assessment by the executive of how the board regards his/her contribution to the organization. Sometimes executive recruiters suggest that boards offer potential candidates a contract to effectively recruit and retain highly talented executives. Experts mostly believe that third parties should be consulted when the executive and board conduct their negotiations. Attorneys, experienced executive recruiters, or other consultants can suggest additional points for consideration and clarify issues that may not be addressed in standard agreements.

Components of executive employment contracts include the term, a general description of duties and reporting relationship, and compensation issues. A minimum salary is stipulated, to which additions can be provided based on a regular performance evaluation (at least annually), sign-on bonuses (for the new executive), incentive compensation (which is increasingly being covered in contracts), and deferred compensation (particularly for older executives). A separate letter of agreement between the board chairman and the CEO should spell out specific benefits and perquisites associated with the position. This benefit package should be designed to meet the unique needs of the individual executive.

Termination agreements—agreements about compensation and benefits for the terminated executive—are central elements of an employment contract. Except for intentional illegal misconduct, termination agreements should not include competency clauses because they pose serious problems of definition and lead to lengthy legal battles. Provisions often incorporated in termination clauses include restrictive covenant clauses such as noncompete, confidentiality, and arbitration requirements. In the event these are used, they should not impose undue hardship on the executive, such as forcing him/her to stay at the hospital or else leave the area. If possible, restrictive clauses should not extend longer than the severance pay period.

The severance clause specifies what is to be paid to the terminated executive. The period of severance payment should be at least 12 months. The amount of severance should reflect the risks and challenges of the position and the possible difficulty the terminated executive will face in finding a comparable position. In addition, any termination arrangement should include executive outplacement assistance, the purpose of which is to assist in transition from one leadership position to another.

Epilogue

EMPLOYMENT CONTRACTS for healthcare executives promote organizational change. This finding has been borne out by searching
the literature and by interviewing attorneys, executive recruiters, compensation consultants, and executives themselves. Given
the uncertainty and resistance that efforts to change organizations—especially ones so complex as those that deliver healthcare
services—a contract that facilitates more decisive leadership benefits the employer and the executive employee.

In the first decade of this century, there are no signs that the
healthcare environment has lost any of its turbulence. Healthcare
leaders continue to face serious financial challenges and threats to
organizational continuity. As has long been the case, advancing the
development of their organizations may require executives to place
the institutions at risk. A newer leadership challenge for boards and
executives is the governmental and public scrutiny surrounding tax
exempt status, adequacy of community benefit, and appropriate-
ness of executive compensation in not-for-profit institutions. Taken
together, these challenges argue for providing enabling mechanisms,
such as contracts, to promote necessary organizational change.

How does the executive employment contract help? First, it
specifies the accountabilities of the position. It shows what the
board expects of the CEO. Second, the contract facilitates the

executive's work efforts for the institution's best interest, which may include forming mergers and other partnerships in which the CEO's position may be eliminated. Thus, the contract is not a guarantee of tenure; instead, it is a mechanism to ensure that the CEO acts in the institution's best interest. Third, in today's integrated environment, executives need to include physicians in decision making. The contract may assist executives to accomodate the shifting power relationships in healthcare organizations as they promote collaboration with physicians.

Overall then, environmental changes have increased the utility of executive employment contracts. From the hospital's perspective, the CEO with a contract can be expected to function more effectively as a decision maker, as a policy advocate, and in leadership exchanges with board members, physicians, providers, payers, and others in the community. Boards that offer contracts are able to attract top management talent. Indeed, the contract itself symbolizes the board's confidence in the CEO they have appointed.

For the executive, a contract affords familiarity with the board's expectations and provides the benefit of a rigorous and regular evaluation. Moreover, it affords the CEO some compensation if, for any reason, the board and the CEO can no longer maintain a productive working partnership. Nevertheless, raising the issue of a contract may work against a CEO with whom the board is only marginally satisfied. Also, a contract may give a CEO a false sense of security. Increasingly, to attract other high-performing CEO executives, contracts are being offered with the expectation that similar advantages will accrue to the organization and the executives themselves.

In sum, for personal, organizational, and community reasons, executive employment contracts for hospital CEOs appear to have merit. Personally, CEOs may be more likely to realize their career objectives for personal growth and development. Organizations benefit from attracting and retaining strong, innovative executives. And, finally, contracts may help communities establish innovative health partnerships that open access to newer technology and improve delivery of care.

2008 ACHE Employment Survey

IN SPRING 2008, ACHE surveyed 981 hospital CEO affiliates regarding executive employment contracts for themselves and their management staff. Responses were received from 505 (52 percent) of those individuals.

Among the hospital CEOs who responded to the survey, 56 percent indicated that they currently have an employment contract. A significantly higher proportion of CEOs in freestanding hospitals (75 percent) reported having a contract than CEOs in system hospitals (32 percent).

Exhibit A.1 Attitudes Toward Executive Employment Contracts Among Hospital CEOs* Who Have an Employment Contract

	% Disagree or Strongly Disagree	% Neutral	% Agree or Strongly Agree
What I value most about the contract is knowing that I have adequate protection in the event of involuntary separation.	6	7	87
The contract's "noncompete" requirements are reasonable (excluding "does not apply" responses).	8	17	75

(continued)

Exhibit A.1 (*continued*)

	% Disagree or Strongly Disagree	% Neutral	% Agree or Strongly Agree
The contract gives me security when board/corporate office leadership changes.	11	16	74
The contract protects me adequately in the event of a change in control.	10	15	74
Knowing that I have a contract helps me take necessary risks in my role as CEO.	8	19	73
My contract is very specific about what is expected of me as CEO.	18	32	50
With a contract, I feel greater freedom to implement new programs and services.	20	30	49
What's most important is knowing my job is secure for the next few years.	19	31	49
With a contract I can exert more forceful leadership with the board/corporate office.	21	34	45
I prefer a contract that specifically states what is expected of me to a more general one.	29	27	44
A contract communicates to the medical staff that I have the strong backing of the board/corporate office.	28	30	42

*Based on a five-point scale from "strongly disagree" to "strongly agree."

Source: American College of Healthcare Executives. 2008. "CEOs' Attitudes about Contracts for Themselves and Their Management Team Members," CEO Circle White Paper, Summer 2008.

Terms of Employment for Healthcare Executives
American College of Healthcare Executives
Professional Policy Statement

November 2008 (revised)

STATEMENT OF THE ISSUE

LEADING A SUCCESSFUL HEALTHCARE ORGANIZATION has become increasingly challenging and fraught with risk. In response to changing external demands and mounting internal pressures, healthcare organizations require a senior management team whose members can confidently assume prudent risks, embrace opportunities involving significant change, and lead with decisiveness.

The American College of Healthcare Executives (ACHE) recognizes that providing executive employment contracts for the chief executive officer and other key members of senior management is one tool that a governing board can use to retain and recruit capable and unwavering leadership during such an era of change and challenge. The provisions of an executive employment contract also can reduce legal and market risks to the organization when a senior executive leaves.

The hospital CEO turnover rate, ranging between 14 and 16 percent between 2002 and 2007, is one indication of the volatility resulting from the challenges faced by leaders of healthcare organizations. Given the link that exists between leadership continuity and overall organizational performance, it is in the best interests of both the organization and the community it serves to provide

CEOs and other appropriate senior-level executives with well-defined protections. Ensuring income continuity and a reasonable transition process encourages prudent decision making based on mutually understood priorities and demonstrates a commitment to equitable and well-respected employment practices.

POLICY POSITION

ACHE believes executive employment contracts for chief executive officers and other appropriate senior executives benefit organizations and individuals. Executive employment contracts allow organizations to clearly establish the executive's leadership role, provide conditions for an orderly transition with continued governance focus on continuity of operations if termination occurs, and provide a measure of income security for executives. As a result, executive employment contracts can foster greater innovation and acceptance of the risks associated with leading complex organizations during a period of significant change.

ACHE encourages all healthcare organizations to wholeheartedly pursue the following actions:

- Provide executive employment contracts or letters of agreement to their chief executive officers with a goal of establishing conditions conducive to the exercise of strong and innovative CEO leadership.
- Provide executive employment contracts or letters of agreement to all other appropriate senior-level executives to similarly promote strong and innovative leadership.
- Provide a balanced contract, including both organizational and individual protections, with clauses addressing issues such as compensation, benefits, perquisites, professional development, participation in outside activities (e.g., serving on external boards), confidentiality and ethical behavior, and potential prohibitions covering a departing executive

accepting employment with a competitor or recruiting other key employees from the organization.

- Provide CEOs with the contractual assurance of a minimum of one year's total compensation (salary plus all benefits that can be legally continued) upon termination without cause with continuation of compensation for up to another six months if needed to find another comparable position.
- Provide other appropriate senior-level executives with a minimum of six months' total compensation (salary plus all benefits that can be legally continued) upon termination without cause with continuation of compensation for up to another six months if needed to find another comparable position.
- Provide chief executive officers and other appropriate senior-level executives with comprehensive outplacement services in the event of termination, including assistance in career plan development and job-search assistance.

Providing an executive employment contract to the CEO and other senior executives can be a valuable tool for the board of a hospital or health system. In addition to retaining and recruiting leaders, a contract can help establish an environment in which executives feel empowered to undertake needed innovation and reasonable risks to further the achievement of the organization's mission.

REFERENCES

American College of Healthcare Executives. 2008. "Hospital CEO Turnover 1981–2007." [Online article; retrieved 9/16/08.] www.ache.org/PUBS/research/ceoturnover.cfm.

American College of Healthcare Executives. 2002. *Contracts for Healthcare Executives*, 4th edition. Chicago: Health Administration Press.

Additional information on contracts and contract provisions is available in the "Career Services for Affiliates" section of ache.org.

Approved by the Board of Governors of the American College of Healthcare Executives on November 10, 2008.

Evaluating the Performance of the Hospital or Health System CEO
American College of Healthcare Executives Professional Policy Statement

November 2008 (revised)

STATEMENT OF THE ISSUE

Board evaluation of the hospital or health system chief executive officer is an important way to ensure that the CEO understands the board's performance expectations and receives feedback on the board's assessment of progress toward their attainment. In an environment characterized by unprecedented challenges, risks, and uncertainty, CEOs are faced with new and more complex responsibilities. Concurrently, public and regulatory expectations demand that boards demonstrate higher levels of accountability for core responsibilities such as the evaluation of leadership performance. As a result, the board's evaluation of the CEO requires a well-designed, ongoing system for measuring leadership effectiveness and the attainment of established objectives.

POLICY POSITION

The American College of Healthcare Executives believes the board of a hospital or health system should evaluate the performance of its chief executive officer using the following principles:

- The evaluation should include an assessment of the CEO's performance on core leadership responsibilities as established by the CEO's job description. In addition, prior to the start of the operating year the board should establish a balanced set of well-defined, measurable objectives to be used in evaluating CEO performance.
- Certain leadership traits such as judgment and diplomacy may require subjective assessment by the board. To the greatest extent feasible the board should evaluate the CEO's performance based on relevant, multifaceted data relating to performance on community, organizational and individual professional objectives:
  - Community objectives might include initiatives such as addressing access to prenatal care, smoking cessation, early detection of chronic diseases, efforts to educate the community about important health issues, etc.
  - Organizational objectives might include a range of quality, patient safety, operational effectiveness, employee engagement, marketplace performance, financial, and satisfaction indicators.
  - Individual professional objectives might include establishing effective board, medical staff, and community relationships; promoting ethical behavior; and continuing professional development by participating in appropriate learning and credentialing activities.
- Providing evaluative feedback for the CEO should be a formal, continuous process involving the board chair or other appropriate board member who confers with the CEO regularly. The board as a whole also should participate by providing feedback through a formal process that collects and collates individual board member assessments of CEO performance, which are considered through documented discussion. The evaluation process should culminate in a formal, annual performance review. Such a continuous evaluation process facilitates timely, meaningful

feedback on many aspects of operations and addresses any misunderstandings or gaps in expectations.

- The evaluation process should enhance the working relationship and information-sharing between the CEO and the board, rather than be a one-directional process. A current CEO position description can be a valuable resource to help guide an effective review.
- If the board determines compensation in association with the formal performance review, then changes in compensation should take into account the full range of objectives established as part of the review process and should not be based solely on financial results.
- As an adjunct to the CEO evaluation process, a board self-evaluation process should be considered. Self evaluations of the full board and individual members constitute important enhancements to the CEO performance evaluation process by assessing the extent to which board members perceive the board provides clear expectations and effective guidance and feedback to the CEO throughout the year.

One of the most important responsibilities of a hospital or health system's board is the development and implementation of a documented, well-designed, ongoing process for providing feedback to the CEO and measuring progress on achieving objectives. Such a process increases communication between the board and the CEO, which ultimately improves the functioning of the organization.

REFERENCE

American College of Healthcare Executives. 2003. *Evaluating the Performance of the Hospital CEO*, 3rd edition. Chicago: Health Administration Press.

Approved by the Board of Governors of the American College of Healthcare Executives on November 10, 2008.

Model Contracts

Appendixes D and E are model contracts between hospitals and their CEOs and senior executives. They are only intended to serve as guides for negotiation between the executive and his or her organization. The details of each contract will vary depending on the institution's situation, the needs and desires of the executive and his or her board, and the laws of the state in which the institution is located. As with any contractual arrangement, the advice of legal, financial, and benefits consultants should be sought before finalizing the agreement.

Model Chief Executive Officer Employment Contract (Long Form)

This agreement, made and effective as of the ____ day of _____, 20XX, between [name of Healthcare Organization], a corporation and [name of CEO].

WHEREAS, the Healthcare Organization desires to secure the services of the CEO and the CEO desires to accept such employment.

NOW THEREFORE, in consideration of the mutual covenants contained in this Agreement, and intending to be legally bound, the Healthcare Organization and the CEO agree as follows:

1.   The CEO will render full-time services to the Healthcare Organization in the capacity of Chief Executive Officer of the corporation. The CEO will at all times, faithfully, industriously and to the best the CEO's ability, perform all duties that may be required of him by virtue of his position as Chief Executive Officer and all duties set forth in Healthcare Organization bylaws and in policy statements of the Board. It is understood that these duties shall be substantially the same as those of a chief executive officer of a business corporation. The CEO shall have and shall perform any special duties assigned or delegated to him by the Board.

2. In consideration for these services as Chief Executive Officer, the Healthcare Organization agrees to pay the CEO a base salary of $_____ per annum or such higher figure as shall be agreed upon at an annual review of his compensation and performance by the Board. This annual review shall occur three months prior to the end of each year of the contract for the express purpose of considering increments. Salary shall be payable in accordance with the payroll policies of the Healthcare Organization. The CEO may elect to defer such portion of his salary to the extent permitted by law in accordance with policies established by the Healthcare Organization. If the employer is required to prepare any restatement of Medicare Cost reports, due to the material noncompliance of the Executive, which comes as a result of his or her misconduct related to any reporting requirement under the Medicare laws, the Executive shall reimburse the Employer for any bonus or other incentive-based compensation received from the Employer during the 12-month period following the first filing with Medicare.

3. (a) The CEO shall be entitled to _____ days of paid time off for vacation and sick leave each year, to be taken at times agreed upon by the Chairman of the Board.

    (b) In the event of a single period of prolonged inability to work due to the results of a sickness or an injury, the CEO will be compensated at his full rate of pay for at least _____ months from the date of the sickness or injury.

    (c) In addition, the CEO will be permitted to be absent from the Healthcare Organization during working days to attend business and educational meetings and to attend to such outside duties in the healthcare field as have been agreed upon by the Chairman of the Board. Attendance at such approved meetings and accomplishment of approved professional duties shall be fully compensated service time and shall not be considered vacation time. The Healthcare Organization shall reimburse the CEO for all expenses incurred by the CEO incident to attendance at approved professional meetings, and such entertainment expenses incurred by the CEO in furtherance of the Healthcare Organization's interests; provided, however, that such reimbursement is approved by the Chairman of the Board.

(d)   In addition, the CEO shall be entitled to all other fringe benefits to which all other employees of the Healthcare Organization are entitled.

4.   The Healthcare Organization agrees to pay dues to professional associations and societies and to such service organizations and clubs of which the CEO is a member, approved by the Chairman of the Board as being in the best interests of the Healthcare Organization.

5.   The Healthcare Organization also agrees to:

(a)   insure the CEO under its general liability insurance policy for all acts done by him in good faith as Chief Executive Officer throughout the term of this contract;

(b)   provide, throughout the term of this contract, a group life insurance policy for the CEO in an amount equivalent to $_____, payable to the beneficiary of his choice;

(c)   provide comprehensive health and major medical insurance for the CEO and his family;

(d)   purchase travel accident insurance covering the CEO in the sum of $_____;

(e)   furnish, for the use of the CEO, an automobile, leased or purchased at the beginning of alternate fiscal years, and reimburse him for expenses of its operation; and

(f)   contribute on behalf of the CEO to a retirement plan qualified under the Internal Revenue Code, at the rate of $_____ per month.

6.   The Board may, in its discretion, terminate this Agreement and the CEO's duties hereunder. Such action shall require a majority vote of the entire Board and become effective upon written notice to the CEO or at such later time as may be specified in said notice. After such termination, the Healthcare Organization shall continue to pay the CEO's then monthly base salary for the month in which his duties were terminated and for 24 consecutive months thereafter as an agreed upon severance payment. During this period, the CEO shall not be required to perform any duties for the Healthcare Organization or come to the Healthcare Organization. Neither shall the fact that the CEO seeks, accepts, and undertakes other employment during this period affect such payments. Also, for the period during which such payments are being made, the Healthcare Organization agrees to keep the CEO's group life, health, and major medical insurance coverage paid up and in effect and the CEO shall be entitled to outplacement services offered by the Healthcare Organization. The severance arrangements described in this paragraph will not be payable in the event that the CEO's employment is terminated due to the fact that the CEO has been charged with any felony criminal offense, or any misdemeanor criminal offense related to substance abuse, healthcare fraud or abuse, violent crimes, sexual misconduct, crimes involving children or the operation of the Healthcare Organization, or has been excluded from Medicare, Medicaid, or any other Federal Healthcare Program.

7.   Should the Board in its discretion change the CEO's duties or authority so it can reasonably be found that the CEO is no longer performing as the Chief Executive Officer of the Healthcare Organization and/or its parent corporation, the CEO shall have the right, within 90 days of such event, in his complete discretion, to terminate this contract by written notice delivered to the Chairman of the Board. Upon such termination, the CEO shall be entitled to the

severance payment described in Paragraph 6, in accordance with the same terms of that Paragraph.

8. If the Healthcare Organization is merged, sold, or closed, the CEO may, at the CEO's discretion, terminate this Agreement or be retained as President of the Healthcare Organization, or any successor corporation to or holding company of the Healthcare Organization. If the CEO elects to terminate his employment at such time, he shall be entitled to the same severance arrangement as would be applicable under Paragraph 6 if the Healthcare Organization had terminated his employment at such time. Any election to terminate employment under this Paragraph must be made prior to the Healthcare Organization's merger, sale or closure, as applicable. If the CEO elects to continue to be employed by the Healthcare Organization or its successor organization, all of the terms and conditions of this Agreement shall remain in effect. The Healthcare Organization agrees that neither it nor its present or any future holding company shall enter into any agreement that would negate or contradict the provisions of this Agreement.

9. Should the CEO in his discretion elect to terminate this contract for any other reason than as stated in Paragraph 7 or 8, he shall give the Board 90 days written notice of his decision to terminate. At the end of the 90 days, all rights, duties and obligations of both parties to the contract shall cease and the CEO will not be entitled to severance benefits.

10. If an event described in Paragraphs 6, 7, or 8 occurs and the CEO accepts any of the severance benefits or payments described therein, the CEO shall to the extent not prohibited by law be deemed to voluntarily release and forever discharge the Healthcare Organization and its officers, directors, employees, agents, and related corporations and their successors and assigns, both individually and collectively and in their official capacities (hereinafter referred to collectively as "Releasees"), from

any and all liability arising out of employment and/or the cessation of said employment. Nothing contained in this paragraph shall prevent the CEO from bringing an action to enforce the terms of this Agreement.

11. The CEO shall maintain confidentiality with respect to information that he receives in the course of his employment and not disclose any such information. The CEO shall not, either during the term of employment or thereafter, use or permit the use of any information of, or relating to the Healthcare Organization in connection with any activity or business and shall not divulge such information to any person, firm, or corporation whatsoever, except as may be necessary in the performance of his duties hereunder or as may be required by law or legal process.

12. During the term of this employment and during the 24 month period following termination of his employment, the CEO shall not directly own, manage, operate, join, control, or participate in or be connected with, as an officer, employee, partner, stockholder, or otherwise, any other hospital, medical clinic, integrated delivery system, health maintenance organization, or related business, partnership, firm, or corporation (all of which hereinafter are referred to as "entity") that is at the time engaged principally or significantly in a business that is, directly or indirectly, at the time in competition with the business of the Healthcare Organization within the service area of the Healthcare Organization. The service area is defined as [DESCRIBE BY COUNTIES, ZIP CODES, A MILEAGE RADIUS, ETC.]. Nothing herein shall prohibit the CEO from acquiring or holding any issue of stock or securities of any entity that has any securities listed on a national securities exchange or quoted in a daily listing of over-the-counter market securities, provided that at any one time the CEO and members of the CEO's immediate family do not own more than 1 percent of

any voting securities of any such entity. This covenant shall be construed as an agreement independent of any other provision of this Agreement, and the existence of any claim or cause of action, whether predicated on this Agreement or otherwise, shall not constitute a defense to the enforcement by the Healthcare Organization of this covenant. In the event of actual or threatened breach by the CEO of this provision, the Healthcare Organization shall be entitled to an injunction restraining the CEO from violation or further violation of the terms thereof.

13.   The CEO shall not directly or indirectly through his own efforts, or otherwise, during the term of this Agreement, and for a period of 24 months thereafter, employ, solicit to employ, or otherwise contract with, or in any way retain the services of any employee or former employee of the Healthcare Organization, if such individual has provided professional or support services to the Healthcare Organization at any time during this Agreement without the express written consent of the Healthcare Organization. The CEO will not interfere with the relationship of the Healthcare Organization and any of its employees and the CEO will not attempt to divert from the Healthcare Organization any business in which the Healthcare Organization has been actively engaged during his employment.

14.   Terms of a new contract shall be completed, or the decision made not to negotiate a new contract made, not later than the end of the tenth month. This contract and all its terms and conditions shall continue in effect until terminated.

15.   This contract constitutes the entire agreement between the parties and contains all the agreements between them with respect to the subject matter hereof. It also supersedes any and all other agreements or contracts, either oral or written, between the parties with respect to the subject matter hereof.

16.   Except as otherwise specifically provided, the terms and conditions of this contract may be amended at any time

by mutual agreement of the parties, provided that before any amendment shall be valid or effective it shall have been reduced to writing and signed by the Chairman of the Board and the CEO.

17. The invalidity or unenforceability of any particular provision of this contract shall not affect its other provisions, and this contract shall be construed in all respects as if such invalid or unenforceable provision had been omitted.

18. This agreement shall be binding upon the Healthcare Organization, its successors and assigns, including, without limitation, any corporation into which the Healthcare Organization may be merged or by which it may be acquired, and shall inure to the benefit of the CEO, his administrators, executors, legatees, heirs and assigns.

19. This agreement shall be construed and enforced under and in accordance with the laws of the State of _____.

20. Any controversy, dispute or disagreement arising out of or relating to this Agreement, or the breach thereof, shall be settled by arbitration, which shall be conducted in _____, _____ in accordance with the American Health Lawyers Association Alternative Dispute Resolution Service Rules of Procedure for Arbitration, and judgment on the award rendered by the arbitrator may be entered in any court having jurisdiction thereof.

This contract signed this _____ day of _____, 20XX.

(NAME OF HEALTHCARE ORGANIZATION)

WITNESS: _____ BY: _____
(Board Chair)

WITNESS: _____ BY: _____
(Name of CEO)

Annotations to
Chief Executive Officer Contract
(Long Form)

This contract is the "long form" CEO contract. It is somewhat more formal than the letter of agreement and specifically lays out some of the minimal benefits that a CEO should receive. Its formality and extensiveness make it more applicable as part of the negotiations for a new relationship than as a contract proposed during an existing one. It should be examined so that the items covered are raised in the negotiations rather than for the exact benefit and salary structure stated. Some benefits will be agreed upon and some not. That is the purpose of a contract negotiation.

PARAGRAPH 1

This paragraph sets forth the duties of the Chief Executive Officer in very general terms. The specific duties of the CEO are not spelled out in the contract itself for two reasons. First, since the CEO should be involved in virtually every area of hospital operations, he must not be hamstrung by a limited "laundry list" of duties that narrowly circumscribe the scope of his responsibility. Such lists relegate the CEO to the status of a "hired hand." In addition, since the duties of the CEO constantly change as the organization changes, it is unwise to lock him and the Healthcare Organization into a set routine from the start. The contract likens the CEO's role to that of a CEO in a business corporation to underscore the broad responsibility entrusted with him.

PARAGRAPH 2

This paragraph contains the financial terms of the contract, specifically, the CEO's salary. An annual figure is inserted in the first blank, while his monthly pay rate should be included in the second blank. The latter, of course, can be a weekly or bimonthly rate, depending on how the hospital or executive payroll is so structured. After each annual salary review, the CEO's salary will presumably increase. New salary levels should be contained in a letter to the CEO from the Board Chairman, which will become incorporated into the initial contract. By the contract language the CEO is also permitted the discretion to direct that a portion of his salary go into tax shelters as deferred income to the extent permitted by law.

PARAGRAPH 3

This paragraph deals in general with compensation for time spent by the CEO away from the hospital, including vacation, sick leave and out-of-hospital business. An alternative to laying these benefits out in the contract is to include them in a separate letter agreement.

Subparagraph 3(a) deals with vacation time for the CEO. Vacation time is compensated at the CEO's full rate, and can be accumulated over the life of the contract.

Subparagraph 3(b) deals with sick leave in a similar fashion except that, unlike vacation time, it cannot be accumulated.

Subparagraph 3(c) deals with disability payments in the event of a major sickness or injury to the CEO. It can take the place of or supplement any disability insurance policy that the CEO may have in effect.

Subparagraph 3(d) permits the CEO to attend professional or hospital association meetings. The meetings to be attended should be agreed to in advance, or expense accounts approved after the fact by the Chairman of the Board. According to this clause, the CEO is entitled to reimbursement for all his expenses and for his full salary while in attendance at these meetings. Also, the travel expenses of the CEO's spouse and any necessary business entertainment expenses are also paid for. It should be stressed that the Chairman of the Board should approve all expense accounts of the CEO, for the CEO's own protection.

PARAGRAPH 4

The CEO's dues for professional associations, service organizations, or clubs that he belongs to are paid for by the Healthcare Organization, so long as his membership in them is reasonably related to the interests of the Healthcare Organization. It should not be necessary that these be approved in advance, but the Chairman of the Board should approve what organizations are joined by the CEO.

PARAGRAPH 5

Subparagraph 5(a) requires the Healthcare Organization to include for coverage the CEO under its general liability insurance policy for any acts done by him in good faith during the course of his duties. This is absolutely essential since CEOs are very often named in lawsuits by patients alleging negligence or by physicians alleging that a denial or termination of medical staff appointment was improper. The Healthcare Organization must protect the CEO if he is to carry out his duties innovatively, aggressively, and effectively.

The fringe benefit described in subparagraph 5(b) provides the CEO with a group life insurance policy, paid for by the Healthcare Organization. Of course, the CEO may name the beneficiaries of this policy. Subparagraphs 5(c) and (d), respectively, provide for comprehensive health insurance and travel accident insurance paid for by the Healthcare Organization. The health insurance package may be with Blue Cross/Blue Shield, a commercial carrier, or the Healthcare Organization's own self-insurance mechanism.

Subparagraph 5(e) provides for an automobile to be used by the CEO, the expenses of which are to be borne by the Healthcare Organization. Finally, subparagraph 5(f) permits payments into a retirement plan which are over and above the CEO's base of salary.

PARAGRAPH 6

This clause is commonly referred to as the termination provision. It is by far the most important part of the Contract. In the event that a majority of the Board decides the services of the CEO are no longer required, for whatever reason, the contract is terminated. However, the CEO will still be entitled to a stated amount of salary even though he or she is no longer working for the Healthcare Organization. Also, the CEO's group life and health insurance benefits continue. Outplacement services are also made available. The exact number of months of severance pay to which the CEO is entitled is of course the subject of negotiation. The figure determined upon should accurately reflect the risks and challenges of the position.

However, this provision relieves the Healthcare Organization from its obligation to pay the severance arrangements in the event that the CEO's employment is terminated due to the CEO being charged with a criminal offense.

The purpose of this clause is to protect the CEO from threats of termination aimed at making him act in his position with unnecessary caution. It is in the interest of the Board, the Healthcare Organization, and the patients. The CEO must be able to exercise his authority to the fullest extent possible. He must also be able to make hard decisions without fear that his job may be in jeopardy simply because someone on the Board or the medical staff did not like the choices he has made.

As an alternative to laying these benefits out in the contract is to include them in a separate agreement. See Appendix A for a model separation agreement.

PARAGRAPH 7

This paragraph is similar to Paragraph 6, except that it comes into play in the event that the Board substantially changes the duties of the CEO, either by appointing another officer with similar duties or by restricting the authority of the existing CEO. This would be one way to avoid the applicability of the severance provisions of Paragraph 6. As in the case of Paragraph 6, the CEO will be entitled to full salary plus group life and health insurance benefits for two years after termination.

PARAGRAPH 8

This paragraph provides for severance payments in the event of merger or closure of the Healthcare Organization.

PARAGRAPH 9

This clause allows the CEO to voluntarily terminate the employment relationship, but if he does, no severance payment is made.

PARAGRAPH 10

This paragraph protects the Healthcare Organization from needless future litigation by the CEO if the CEO accepts the severance benefits. This allows the Healthcare Organization to conduct its business relationship with the CEO without unnecessary caution. It is in the interest of the Board, the Healthcare Organization, and the patients. This waiver will be enforced to the maximum extent allowable by law.

PARAGRAPH 11

This provision protects the Healthcare Organization from disclosure of confidential information by the CEO during and after his term of employment with the Healthcare Organization. An employment contract with a key executive should contain a provision that prohibits the employee from disclosing to outsiders confidential information acquired by the employee during his term of employment without the express written permission of the employer. This provision should describe the applicable information so as to put the employee on notice as to what constitutes confidential information.

PARAGRAPH 12

An employment contract with an executive employee typically contains a covenant by the employee not to compete with the employer during the term of the contract and for a specified period of time following termination of employment. The covenant is essential to the employer in order to prevent the employee from dealing with the employer's customers or otherwise engaging in competitive activities with the employer immediately following his termination of employment so as to cause material adverse financial consequences to the business of the employer.

Restrictive employment covenants have generally been held to be valid where the restraint imposed on the employee is no greater than necessary to protect the legitimate business interests of the employer, and where neither the hardship to the employee nor the likely injury to the public outweighs the employer's need for protection. Thus, a covenant not to compete is usually upheld if it is clearly and reasonably limited as to time and area, and does not extend beyond the duration and geographical scope necessary for the protection of the employer. It should be noted that such restrictive covenants are unenforceable in some states.

PARAGRAPH 13

This provision prevents the CEO whose employment at the Healthcare Organization has been terminated for whatever reason from recruiting other key executives to leave the Healthcare Organization and join him in independent ventures excluding the Healthcare Organization's involvement.

PARAGRAPH 14

This paragraph makes it simple for the Healthcare Organization and the CEO to continue the agreement beyond its initial term by signing a simple letter of agreement as an extension. The letter need only state that the initial contract has been extended for another specified period and set out the CEO's new salary. All of the initial provisions and benefits continue in force during the extension.

PARAGRAPH 15

This is a standard clause that appears in most contracts. It states that this particular contract embodies total agreement of the parties and supersedes any previous contract, in response to the so-called "parole evidence rule" of contract law. It eliminates any questions there may be as to the subject matter contained in the contract.

PARAGRAPH 16

This provision requires that any amendments to the contract be stated in writing. This prevents either side from claiming that an "oral understanding" superseded some portion of this contract. It is technically referred to as a "no oral modification" or NOM clause.

PARAGRAPH 17

This is known technically as a "savings clause." In the event that any portion of the contract is declared invalid or unenforceable by a court, the rest of the contract still remains in effect. The contract can therefore not be terminated on a "technicality."

PARAGRAPH 18

This paragraph keeps the contract in force even though the hospital may change its corporate structure or be sold to another owner. It also provides that any benefits provided under the contract, such as life or accident insurance, that survive the CEO upon his death, inure to the benefit of his estate or heirs.

PARAGRAPH 19

This clause stipulates what law applies to the contract. This is especially useful in hospitals near state lines. The law governing the contract should always be that of the state in which the hospital is located.

The execution of the contract should be authorized by the Board. It should be signed by the Chairman of the Board and the CEO, and should be witnessed by two individuals who are not on the Board and who are not members of the CEO's family. It should be filed along with other essential corporate documents. A copy should be given to the CEO. Needless to say, the terms of the contract, especially those relating to salary levels, fringe benefits and termination, should be treated as confidential.

Model Letter of Agreement for Chief Executive Officer

Dear _____:

[name of Healthcare Organization] desires to secure your services as Chief Executive Officer of [name of Healthcare Organization] and all of its related corporations (hereinafter collectively referred to as "the Employer"), subject to the bylaws of the Employer and the policies of its Board. It is understood that you shall have full authority for the executive management of the organization, subject to the bylaws of the Employer and the policies of its Board. Therefore, in consideration of the mutual covenants contained in this letter, the following provisions will evidence the terms and conditions of such employment, to which both you and the Employer will be legally bound.

1. For your services, the Employer agrees to pay you a base salary, with fringe benefits and the opportunity to earn incentive compensation, as set forth on the attached Exhibit for a one-year period ending on _____. Your performance and compensation shall be reviewed on an annual basis by the Executive Compensation Committee of the Board pursuant to the Executive Compensation Policy and adjusted as approved by that Committee and ratified by the Board. Your base

salary will be paid in accordance with the normal payroll policies of the Employer.

2. The Board may, in its discretion, terminate your employment at any time, and for any reason, by giving written notice to you. Upon such termination, all rights, duties, and obligations of both parties shall cease, except that the Employer shall continue to pay you your then monthly base salary and maintain your health insurance benefits in effect for a period of 24 months (including the month in which termination occurred) as an agreed-upon severance payment, subject to your executing a written separation agreement which shall provide for such salary and benefit continuation and contain terms and conditions normally found in such agreements, including a mutual release of liability. The severance payments described in this paragraph will not be payable in the event that your employment is terminated due to the fact that you have been charged with any felony, or any misdemeanor criminal offense related to substance abuse, healthcare fraud or abuse, violent crimes, sexual misconduct, or crimes involving children or the operations of the Employer.

3. Should the Board, in its discretion, change your duties or authority so it can reasonably be found that you are no longer performing as the Chief Executive Officer of the Employer and/or its parent corporation, you shall have the right, within 90 days of such event, to terminate your employment by written notice delivered to the Chairman of the Board. Upon such termination, you shall be entitled to the severance payments described in the preceding paragraph.

4. If the Employer or its holding company is merged, sold, or closed, or if control of the Employer or its holding company is transferred to a different corporation, you may at your discretion terminate your employment or be

retained as Chief Executive Officer of the Employer, or any successor corporation to, or the holding company of, the Employer. If you elect to terminate your employment at such time, you shall be entitled to the same severance payments as would be applicable under Paragraph 3 if the Employer had terminated your employment at such time.

i. Any election to terminate employment under this paragraph must be made prior to the Employer's merger, sale, or closure, as applicable.

ii. If you elect to continue to be employed by the Employer or its successor organization, all of the terms and conditions of this Agreement shall remain in effect. The Employer agrees that neither it nor its present, or any future, holding company shall enter into any agreement that would negate or contradict the provisions of this Agreement.

5. You may also terminate your employment at any time, for any other reason, by giving at least 30 days' advance written notice to the Chairman of the Board. If you do, all rights, duties, and obligations of both parties will cease and you will not be entitled to any severance benefits.

6. If an event described in Paragraphs 3, 4, or 5 occurs and you accept any of the severance benefits or payments described therein, you shall be deemed to have voluntarily released and forever discharged the Employer and its officers, directors, employees, agents, and related corporations and their successors and assigns, both individually and collectively and in their official capacities, from any and all liability arising out of your employment and/or the cessation of said employment. Nothing contained in this paragraph shall prevent you from bringing an action to enforce the terms of this Agreement.

7. You acknowledge that, in the course of your employment, you will have access to confidential information and trade secrets of the Employer, including, without limitation,

information and knowledge pertaining to: patients and patient lists, marketing strategies, business plans, managed care or other payor relationships (including but not limited to rate information), medical staff, pending or actual litigation, peer review matters, corporate compliance matters, personnel matters, vendor relationships, and all other confidential or proprietary information (collectively, "Confidential Information"). You agree to maintain confidentiality with respect to Confidential Information that you receive in the course of your employment and shall not disclose any such Confidential Information without the express written permission of the Employer. You shall not, either during the term of employment or thereafter, use or permit the use of any Confidential Information of, or relating to, the Employer in connection with any activity or business and shall not divulge such Confidential Information to any person, firm, or corporation whatsoever, except as may be necessary in the performance of your duties hereunder or as may be required by law or legal process. The obligation of confidentiality imposed by this Paragraph shall not apply to information that becomes generally known to the public through no act of you in breach of this Agreement. Further, in the event of any dispute concerning this Agreement, you may disclose to your attorney such Confidential Information as may be directly relevant to such dispute, or to the court, subject to the terms of a confidentiality agreement, and protective order, reached by the parties and approved by the court.

8. For a period of _____ (_____) months following the termination of your employment, you shall not, unless acting pursuant hereto or with the prior written consent of the Board of the Employer, directly or indirectly, own, manage, operate, finance, join, control, or participate in or be connected with, as an officer, director, employee,

partner, principal, agent, representative, consultant, or otherwise, or use or permit your name to be used in connection with: (i) any other hospital or healthcare facility, health system, or related business that is at the time engaged principally or significantly in a business that is, directly or indirectly, at the time in competition with the business of the Employer and within the service area of the Employer, or (ii) any entity doing business with the Employer within _____ (_____) years of the termination of this Agreement. For purposes of this Paragraph, the geographical service area shall be defined as within (_____) miles of [City], [State]. Notwithstanding the foregoing, Paragraphs 8 and 9 shall not be construed to limit you from engaging in activities on behalf of a multilocational entity to the extent that your duties and responsibilities relate primarily to locations outside of such geographic service area. In addition, you may own up to _____ percent (_____%) of the outstanding stock of public companies without violating this Paragraph.

9. For a period of _____ (_____) months following the termination of your employment, you shall not, unless acting pursuant hereto or with the prior written consent of the Board, directly or indirectly, on your own behalf or as a principal, representative or agent of any person, hospital, healthcare facility, health system, or related business, solicit or induce any employee, contractor or consultant of the Employer to terminate, reduce or otherwise alter his or her relationship with the Employer or to enter into the employment of or a similar relationship with any other hospital, healthcare facility, health system, or related business. You shall not engage in any attempt to divert from the Employer any business in which the Employer was actively engaged during your employment, or made material plans to engage in during or after your employment. Notwithstanding the foregoing, if you are

employed by another entity under circumstances that are not otherwise a violation of Paragraphs 8 or 9, you may employ or solicit contractors or consultants of the Employer to provide Services to your new employer on a non-exclusive basis.

10. You shall devote your full professional time, effort, and attention to this position and shall not be otherwise employed or conduct any other outside business or professional activities while employed by the Employer. You shall refrain from any and all conduct that could in any way damage the reputation of the Employer.

[NAME OF ORGANIZATION]

BY:

Chairman of the Board

I accept the terms and conditions contained in the above letter and intend to be legally bound by them.

-

DATE:

Annotations to
Chief Executive Officer Contract
(Letter Agreement)

INTRODUCTORY PARAGRAPH

This paragraph sets forth the basic terms of the contract. It should be noted, however, that the specific duties of the CEO are not spelled out in the contract itself. This is done for two reasons. First, since the CEO should be involved in virtually every area of Healthcare Organization operations, he must not be limited by a "laundry list" of duties that narrowly circumscribes the scope of his responsibility. Such lists can relegate the CEO to the status of a "hired hand." In addition, since the duties of the CEO constantly change as the Healthcare Organization changes, it is unwise to lock him and the Healthcare Organization into a set routine from the start. The contract likens the CEO's role to that of a CEO in a business corporation to underscore the broad responsibility entrusted to him by the Board.

PARAGRAPH 1

This paragraph sets forth the consideration given the CEO in return for his services and requires the CEO to devote his full professional time to the Healthcare Organization. Experience has led us to the conclusion that it is best that the CEO's actual salary and benefits not be laid out in detail in the letter agreement.

Rather, they should be set forth in a separate letter or document from the Executive Compensation Committee of the Board to the CEO. This letter should be kept strictly confidential to the extent permitted in compliance with legal and IRS reporting requirements. All too often the CEO's salary and benefits will be used by dissident elements on the Board or medical staff as a means of attacking the CEO. Although those benefits may be appropriate for the CEO of a company with a budget of tens or hundreds of millions of dollars, they will not be perceived as such by rank and file Healthcare Organization employees or the news media. A separate document will minimize the risk that this sensitive information will fall into the wrong hands.

After each annual salary review, the CEO's salary will presumably increase. New salary levels should be contained in a letter to the CEO from the Board Chairman, which will become incorporated into the initial contract.

PARAGRAPH 2

This paragraph is commonly referred to as the termination clause. It is by far the most important part of the contract. In the event that a majority of the Board decides the services of the CEO are no longer required, for whatever reason, the contract is terminated. However, the CEO will still be entitled to a stated amount of salary even though he is no longer working for the Healthcare Organization. Also, the CEO's group life and health insurance benefits continue. Outplacement services are also provided. Other benefits may continue as negotiated. The exact number of months of severance pay to which the CEO is entitled is of course the subject of negotiation. The figure determined upon should accurately reflect the risks and challenges of the position, as well as the relative difficulty the CEO will face in finding a comparable position.

However, this provision relieves the Healthcare Organization from its obligation to pay the severance arrangements in the event that the CEO's employment is terminated due to the CEO being charged with a criminal offense.

The purpose of this clause is to protect the CEO from threats of termination aimed at making him act in his position with unnecessary caution. It is in the interest of the Board, the Healthcare Organization, and the patients. The CEO must be able to exercise his authority to the fullest extent possible. He must also be able to make hard decisions without fear that his job may be in jeopardy simply because someone on the board or the medical staff dislikes the choices he has made for reasons unrelated to the best interest of the Healthcare Organization.

PARAGRAPH 3

This paragraph is similar to Paragraph 2, except that it comes into play if the board substantially changes the duties of the CEO, either by appointing another officer with similar duties or by restricting the authority of the existing CEO. This would be one way to avoid the applicability of the termination provisions of Paragraph 2. As in the case of Paragraph 2, the CEO in this case will be entitled to full salary plus group life and health insurance benefits for the number of months specified in Paragraph 2.

PARAGRAPH 4

This paragraph provides for severance payments in the event of merger or closure of the Healthcare Organization.

PARAGRAPH 5

This paragraph is similar to paragraphs 2 and 3 except it comes into effect if the CEO voluntarily terminates his employment, for whatever reason, with the Healthcare Organization. This provision also provides that in this event, the termination agreement does not come into effect and the CEO is not entitled to severance benefits.

PARAGRAPH 6

This paragraph protects the Healthcare Organization from needless future litigation by the CEO if the CEO accepts the severance benefits. This allows the Healthcare Organization to conduct its business relationship with the CEO without unnecessary caution. It is in the interest of the Board, the Healthcare Organization, and the patients.

PARAGRAPH 7

This provision protects the Healthcare Organization from disclosure of confidential information by the CEO during and after his term of employment with the Healthcare Organization. An employment contract with a key executive should contain a provision that prohibits the employee from disclosing to outsiders confidential information acquired by the employee during his term of employment without the express written permission of the employer. This provision should describe the applicable information so as to put the employee on notice as to what constitutes confidential information.

PARAGRAPH 8

An employment contract with an executive employee typically contains a covenant by the employee not to compete with the employer during the term of the contract and for a specified period of time following termination of employment. The covenant is essential to the employer in order to prevent the employee from dealing with the employer's customers or otherwise engaging in competitive activities with the employer immediately following his termination of employment so as to cause material adverse financial consequences to the business of the employer.

Restrictive employment covenants have generally been held to be valid where the restraint imposed on the employee is no greater than necessary to protect the legitimate business interests of the employer, and where neither the hardship to the employee nor the likely injury to the public outweighs the employer's need for protection. Thus, a covenant not to compete is usually upheld if it is clearly and reasonably limited as to time and area and does not extend beyond the duration and geographical scope necessary for the protection of the employer. It should be noted that such restrictive covenants are unenforceable in some states.

PARAGRAPH 9

This provision prevents the CEO, whose employment at the Healthcare Organization has been terminated, for whatever reason, from recruiting other key executives to leave the Healthcare Organization and join him in independent ventures excluding the Healthcare Organization's involvement.

The execution of the contract should be authorized by the Board. It becomes effective when it is signed by the Chairman of the Board and accepted by the CEO, or on some later date agreed upon by the parties. It should be filed along with other essential corporate documents, with a duplicate original given to the CEO. Needless to say, the terms of the contract should be treated as confidential.

PARAGRAPH 10

This paragraph is intended to permit the executive to participate in trade and professional organizations like the AHA, state hospital associations, ACHE, and other outside organizations, so long as they would not damage the reputation of the hospital or health system.

Model Letter of Agreement
for Senior Executives

_____
(Date)

Dear _____:

[name of Healthcare Organization] desires to secure your services as Senior Executive of [specify position]. It is understood that your duties shall be determined from time to time by the Chief Executive Officer of the Healthcare Organization, subject to the bylaws of the Healthcare Organization and the policies of the Board. Therefore, in consideration of the material advantages accruing between the Healthcare Organization and you, as well as the mutual covenants contained in this letter, the following provisions will evidence the terms and conditions of such employment, to which both you and the Healthcare Organization will be legally bound.

1. For your services, the Healthcare Organization agrees to pay you your salary and fringe benefits, as set forth on the attached document, and such higher salary and additional fringe benefits as are mutually agreed upon at an annual review of your compensation by the Chief Executive Officer. Your salary will be paid in accordance with the normal payroll policies of the Healthcare Organization. You shall

devote your full professional time, efforts, and attention to this position and shall not be otherwise employed or conduct any other outside business or professional activities while employed by the Healthcare Organization.

2. The Chief Executive Officer may, in his or her discretion, terminate your employment at any time, and for any reason, by giving written notice to you. Upon such termination, all rights, duties and obligations of both parties shall cease, except that the Healthcare Organization shall continue to pay you your then monthly salary for a period of ___ months (including the month in which termination occurred) as an agreed upon severance payment. During this period, you shall not be required to come to the Healthcare Organization or to perform any duties for the Healthcare Organization. However, if you accept and undertake other employment during this period, the Healthcare Organization shall no longer be required to make such payments. Also, during this period, the Healthcare Organization agrees, at its expense, to keep your life, health, and long-term disability insurance fully in effect, and to provide you with outplacement services. The severance arrangements described in this paragraph will not be payable in the event that your employment is terminated due to the fact that you have been charged with any felony criminal offense, or any misdemeanor criminal offense related to substance abuse or to the operation of the Healthcare Organization.

3. The severance arrangements described in Paragraph 2 shall also be available if the Healthcare Organization shall merge, consolidate, or affiliate with or be sold to another person and as a result you are terminated.

4. You may also terminate your employment at any time, for any reason, by giving at least 30 days advance written notice to the Chief Executive Officer, but if you do, all rights, duties, and obligations of both parties will cease and you will not be entitled to any severance benefits.

5. If an event described in Paragraphs 2 or 3 occurs and you accept any of the severance benefits or payments described therein, you shall be deemed to voluntarily release and forever discharge the Healthcare Organization and its officers, directors, employees, agents, and related corporations and their successors and assigns, both individually and collectively and in their official capacities (hereinafter referred to collectively as "Releasees"), from any and all liability arising out of your employment and/or the cessation of said employment and including, but not limited to, any alleged violation of Title VII of the Civil Rights Act of 1964, the Civil Rights Act of 1866 (42 U.S.C. §1981 et seq.), the Employee Retirement Income Security Act of 1974, the Age Discrimination in Employment Act of 1967, the Fair Labor Standards Act, the National Labor Relations Act, or any other federal, state, or local labor, civil, or human rights law, or any other alleged violation of any local, state, or federal law, regulation, or ordinance, and/or public policy, contract, or tort law having any bearing or relationship whatsoever on the terms and/or conditions of your employment that you ever had, now have, or shall have as of the date of this Agreement. Nothing contained in this Paragraph shall prevent you from bringing an action to enforce the terms of this Agreement.

6. You shall maintain confidentiality with respect to information that you receive in the course of your employment and not disclose any such information. You shall not, either during the term of employment or thereafter, use or permit the use of any information of or relating to the Healthcare Organization in connection with any activity or business and shall not divulge such information to any person, firm, or corporation whatsoever, except as may be necessary in the performance of your duties hereunder or as may be required by law or legal process.

7.   During the term of your employment and during the _____ month period following termination of your employment, you shall not directly own, manage, operate, join, control, or participate in or be connected with, as an officer, employee, partner, stockholder, or otherwise, any other Healthcare Organization, medical clinic, integrated delivery system, health maintenance organization, or related business, partnership, firm, or corporation (all of which hereinafter are referred to as "entity") that is at the time engaged principally or significantly in a business that is, directly or indirectly, at the time in competition with the business of the Healthcare Organization within the service area of the Healthcare Organization. The service area is defined as [describe by counties, zip codes, a mileage radius, etc.]. Nothing herein shall prohibit you from acquiring or holding any issue of stock or securities of any entity that has any securities listed on a national securities exchange or quoted in a daily listing of over-the-counter market securities, provided that at any one time you and members of your immediate family do not own more than 1 percent of any voting securities of any such entity. This covenant shall be construed as an agreement independent of any other provision of this Agreement, and the existence of any claim or cause of action, whether predicated on this Agreement or otherwise, shall not constitute a defense to the enforcement by the Healthcare Organization of this covenant. In the event of actual or threatened breach by you of this provision, the Healthcare Organization shall be entitled to an injunction restraining you from violation or further violation of the terms thereof.

8.   You shall not directly or indirectly through your own efforts, or otherwise, during the term of this Agreement, and for a period of ___ months thereafter, employ, solicit to employ, or otherwise contract with, or in any way retain the services of any employee or former employee of the Healthcare Organization, if such individual has

provided professional or support services to the Healthcare Organization at any time during this Agreement, without the express written consent of the Healthcare Organization. You will not interfere with the relationship of the Healthcare Organization and any of its employees and you will not attempt to divert from the Healthcare Organization any business in which the Healthcare Organization has been actively engaged during your employment.

[NAME OF HEALTHCARE ORGANIZATION]

BY:

President and Chief Executive Officer

I accept the terms and conditions contained in the above letter and intend to be legally bound by them.

Senior Executive

DATE:

Annotations to
Senior Executives' Contract

This contract is designed for Senior Executives at the top level of the management team, such as the Chief Operating Officer, Chief Financial Officer, or Medical Director. It is similar to the model CEO contract in all but a few respects.

First, the CEO (not the Board) negotiates and executes the contract on behalf of the Healthcare Organization. It is essential that the CEO's right to hire and discharge subordinates be unchallenged. Otherwise, his authority and ability to manage will be compromised.

Second, this contract does not provide for severance payments in the event that the Senior Executive's job description or duties change. The CEO must also retain the absolute right to change the duties of his management team if he is to run the institution effectively.

In most other respects, this contract resembles the CEO's and the annotations to the CEO's contract also apply here. However, it would be expected that the salary, benefits, and length of severance payments would be less for a Senior Executive than for a CEO.

Model Separation Agreement

BY AND BETWEEN

[Name of Healthcare Organization], a nonprofit corporation organized under the laws of the State of _____ (hereinafter called the "Employer"),

AND

[Name of Executive], an individual (hereinafter called "Executive").

WITNESSETH:

WHEREAS, the Employer and Executive are parties to an Employment Agreement (the "Agreement") which was entered into on _____, 20___, the terms of which were partially modified by an Executive Severance Benefit Plan (the "Severance Plan") effective _____, 20___; and

WHEREAS, the Employer and Executive wish to set forth the terms of Executive's separation from employment and terminate the Agreement and the Severance Plan as specified herein.

NOW, THEREFORE, in consideration of the mutual covenants herein contained and intending to be legally bound hereby, the parties hereto agree as follows:

1. <u>Termination of Employment.</u>
   (a) Executive shall cease to be employed by the Employer as of the close of business on _____, 20___ (the "Termination Date"). Except as expressly provided herein, the Employment Agreement, the Severance Plan, and all amendments thereto are expressly superseded by this Agreement upon its execution by both parties, and all rights and obligations of both parties pursuant thereto shall cease as of the Termination Date. As of _____, 20___, Executive shall no longer serve as President and Chief Executive Officer of the Employer or of any of its subsidiaries, shall no longer perform any duties, and shall not be authorized to act on behalf of the Employer or of any of its subsidiaries. Executive shall also cease to be an officer and a member of the Board of the Employer and of any other entities controlled by the Employer (collectively "Affiliates") as of the Termination Date.
   (b) Executive hereby expressly agrees that he or she will not disclose the terms of the Separation Agreement to any individual or entity not authorized by the Employer or disparage, malign, or otherwise say or do anything that could adversely affect the reputation or standing of the Employer.

2. <u>Payments and Benefits Upon Termination of Employment.</u>
   (a) Executive shall receive his Base Salary for a period of _____ (_____) months from the Termination Date, in accordance with the Employer's regular payroll practices and procedures, in effect from time to time, for senior management executives. "Base Salary" shall mean the total annual base salary payable to Executive at the rate in effect as of the Termination Date, which was _____ dollars ($_____) per annum. During

this _____ (_____) month period, Executive shall not be required to perform any duties for the Employer or any Affiliate. Neither shall the fact that Executive seeks, accepts, and undertakes other employment during this period affect such payments. In addition, the Employer has arranged for a senior executive outplacement program to assist Executive in securing another position, pursuant to the agreement with _____, which is attached as Exhibit _____.

(b) Executive's benefits listed on Exhibit A shall continue during the period when Executive receives severance pay hereunder to the extent that such continuation is permissible under controlling law (e.g., nondiscrimination or risk of forfeiture limitations) and benefit plan and policy provisions (as reasonably determined by the Employer). If a benefit cannot be continued, the Employer shall be released of its obligation to provide such benefit to Executive, and the Employer shall not be obligated to pay Executive any cash or other benefit in lieu of such noncontinued benefit. If the Employer changes the level of coverage or level of benefits under the plans for active employees during the benefit continuation period, the benefits for Executive shall be similarly modified. Executive shall also be entitled to extend said benefits at his own expense beyond the benefit continuation period as specifically provided for by the federal COBRA statute. Except as listed on Exhibit A, all other benefits shall be discontinued. Executive shall receive such distributions or conversion rights as may be provided for by applicable benefit plans.

(c) Executive shall also receive via direct payroll deposit on _____, 20____ $_____ as compensation for _____ hours of unused paid time off to which Executive is entitled under the employee benefit policies of the Employer.

(d) In accordance with the Employment Agreement, Executive shall be entitled to his share of any performance bonus pursuant to the Annual Incentive Plan for the President and Chief Executive Officer for FYE 20___ prorated to reflect the portion of the fiscal year that Executive was employed (i.e., _____/365, or _____% of Executive's full year share, if any). If the Employer is required to prepare any restatement of Medicare Cost reports, due to the material noncompliance of the Executive, which comes as a result of his or her misconduct related to any reporting requirement under the Medicare laws, the Executive shall reimburse the Employer for any bonus or other incentive-based compensation received from the Employer during the 12-month period following the first filing with Medicare.

(e) Payments to Executive under Sections 2(a), (b), (c), and (d) shall be subject to such withholdings for federal income taxes, Social Security, Medicare, FUTA, state and local income, and other applicable taxes as may be required by law from time to time or higher amounts as may be designated by Executive in accordance with applicable laws or regulations.

3. <u>Company Property</u>.

Executive represents to the Employer that he has turned over to the Employer all cell phones, computers, PDAs, pagers, files, memoranda, records, other documents, keys, keycards, and any other physical or personal property of which he has possession, custody or control, which are the property of the Employer, including the automobile that was leased by the Employer for the Executive's use.

4. <u>Miscellaneous</u>.
   (a) Subject to the non-competition clause contained in Section 6, Executive may seek employment elsewhere as of the Termination Date.
   (b) The Employer will refer letters and phone calls that are personal to Executive to his home phone number and address as noted in his personnel file or to such other forwarding address as Executive may designate in writing.
5. <u>Confidential Information</u>.
   Executive acknowledges that, by reason of his employment by the Employer, Executive has had access to confidential information and trade secrets of the Employer and its Affiliates, including, without limitation, information and knowledge pertaining to patients and patient lists, marketing strategies, business plans, managed care or other payor relationships (including but not limited to rate information), medical staff, pending or actual litigation, peer review matters, corporate compliance matters, personnel matters, vendor relationships, and all other confidential or proprietary information (collectively, "Confidential Information"). Executive agrees to maintain confidentiality with respect to Confidential Information that he received in the course of his employment and shall not disclose any such Confidential Information without the express written permission of the Board of the Employer. Executive shall not use or permit the use of any Confidential Information of or relating to the Employer or any Affiliates in connection with any activity or business and shall not divulge such Confidential Information to any person, firm, or corporation whatsoever, except as may be necessary in the performance of his duties hereunder or as may be required by law or legal process. The obligation of confidentiality imposed by this Section shall not apply to

information that becomes generally known to the public through no act of Executive in breach of this Agreement. Further, in the event of any dispute concerning this Agreement, Executive may disclose to his attorney such Confidential Information as may be directly relevant to such dispute, or to the court subject to the terms of a confidentiality agreement, and protective order, reached by the parties and approved by the court.

6.   Non-Competition.

(a)   For a period of _____ (_____) months following the Termination Date, Executive shall not, unless acting pursuant hereto or with the prior written consent of the Board of the Employer, directly or indirectly own, manage, operate, finance, join, control, or participate in or be connected with, as an officer, director, employee, partner, principal, agent, representative, consultant, or otherwise, or use or permit Executive's name to be used in connection with: (i) any other hospital or healthcare facility, health system, or related business that is at the time engaged principally or significantly in a business that is, directly or indirectly, at the time in competition with the business of the Employer or any Affiliate and within the service area of the Employer or any Affiliate, or (ii) any entity doing business with the Employer or any Affiliate within _____ (_____) years of the termination of this Agreement. For purposes of this Section, the geographical service area shall be defined as within (_____) miles of [City], [State]. Notwithstanding the foregoing, (i) this Section shall not be construed to limit Executive from engaging in activities on behalf of a multilocational entity to the extent that his duties and responsibilities relate primarily to locations outside of such geographic service area, and (ii) Executive may own up to _____ percent (_____%) of the outstanding stock of public companies without violating this Section.

(b) For a period of _____ (_____) months thereafter, Executive shall not, unless acting pursuant hereto or with the prior written consent of the Board, directly or indirectly, on Executive's own behalf or as a principal, representative or agent of any person, hospital, healthcare facility, health system, or related business, solicit or induce any employee, contractor, or consultant of the Employer or any Affiliate to terminate, reduce, or otherwise alter his/her relationship with the Employer or any Affiliate or to enter into the employment of or a similar relationship with any other hospital, healthcare facility, health system, or related business. Executive shall not engage in any attempt to divert from the Employer or its Affiliates any business in which the Employer or its Affiliates were actively engaged during his employment, or made material plans to engage in during or after his employment. Notwithstanding the foregoing, if Executive is employed by another entity under circumstances that are not otherwise a violation of this Section 6, Executive may employ or solicit contractors or consultants of the Employer or its Affiliates to provide Services to Executive's new employer on a nonexclusive basis.

(c) Executive acknowledges that the restrictions contained in this Section 6 are, in view of the nature of the business of the Employer and its Affiliates, reasonable and necessary to protect the legitimate interests of the Employer and Affiliates and that any violation of any provision of this Section 6 will result in irreparable injury to the Employer and its Affiliates. Executive also acknowledges that in the event of any such violation, the Employer and/or its Affiliates shall be entitled to preliminary and permanent injunctive relief, without the necessity of proving actual damages, and to the equitable accounting of all earnings, profits, and other benefits arising from any such violation, which rights shall be cumulative and in addition to any other rights or remedies to which the Employer and/or its Affiliates may be entitled. Executive agrees that in the event of any such violation, an action may be commenced for any such preliminary and permanent injunctive relief and other equitable relief in any federal or state court of competent jurisdiction. Further, Executive hereby waives, to the fullest extent permitted by law, any objection that Executive may now or hereafter have to such jurisdiction or to the laying of the venue of any such suit, action, or proceeding brought in such a court and any claim that such suit, action, or proceeding has been brought in an inconvenient forum.

7. <u>Adequate Consideration</u>.

The Employer and Executive each agree that the consideration set forth in this Separation Agreement is adequate and sufficient consideration to extinguish any right or obligation that either party may have to the other party pursuant to the Employment Agreement. As such, the Employer and Executive each agree not to commence any arbitration, mediation, claim, or proceeding, or any other form of action in law or equity, against each other, arising out of or related to the execution, performance, or termination of Executive's employment and hereby waive all rights to the same.

8. <u>Releases</u>.

(a) The Employer, on behalf of itself and its respective officers, directors, agents, executives, representatives, affiliates, successors, and assigns, hereby agrees to fully release, discharge, and forever hold harmless Executive and his estate, representatives, executors, and heirs from any and all liability or claims (including, but not limited to, claims for damages, punitive damages, costs, or attorneys' fees), whether known or unknown, related to or arising out of the execution or performance of Executive's duties while employed by the Employer, other than intentional wrongful conduct on the part of Executive.

(b)   Executive, on behalf of himself and his estate, representatives, executors and heirs, successors, and assigns, hereby agrees to fully release, discharge, and forever hold harmless the Employer and its officers, trustees, agents, executives, representatives, affiliates, successors and assigns from any and all liability or claims (including, but not limited to, claims for damages, punitive damages, costs, or attorneys' fees), whether known or unknown, related to or arising out of the Employment Agreement, the Severance Plan, any action taken by the same related to Executive's employment with the Employer, the execution of this Agreement or the termination of Executive's employment. Said release shall include, but not be limited to, any claim or action that may now or hereafter be asserted by Executive purporting to be violations of any state or federal statutes such as Title VII of the Civil Rights Act of 1964, the Americans with Disabilities Act, the Family and Medical Leave Act, the Age Discrimination in Employment Act of 1967, [applicable state law], federal or state or common law, or the Constitution of any state or of the United States, and Executive hereby expressly waives any and all legal or equitable remedies which may have been available to him thereunder including, but not limited to, any claim for attorneys' fees.

(c)   The releases set forth in Sections 8(a) and (b) do not preclude Executive from seeking indemnification from any action arising out of the acts or omissions of Executive while he was the Chief Executive Officer of the Employer.

(d) Executive represents that he has provided the Employer with any and all information that he possesses that he reasonably believes might cause the Employer or any of its Affiliates to incur any civil or criminal liability to the state or federal government and, as such, hereby waives any right he may now or hereafter possess to act as a relator in a qui tam suit against the Employer on behalf of the United States and/or the State of _____ under the False Claims Act or any similar federal or state statute and further agrees never to file any such suit.

(e) In the event that Executive or his estate, representatives, heirs, or executors bring any action or claim for any matter subject to the release set forth in this Section, all payments due to Executive hereunder shall cease, and the benefits provided under this Agreement shall be forfeited.

(f) Notwithstanding the above, if any party violates the terms and conditions of this Agreement, the aggrieved party may pursue an appropriate action at law or equity to enforce this Agreement.

(g) The foregoing releases may never be treated as an admission of liability by either party for any purpose.

9. Cooperation in Event of Claims or Investigations; Indemnification; Continued Insurance Coverage.

(a) The parties will fully cooperate with each other in the event that any claims are brought against either or both of them or investigations are instituted by government agencies regarding matters related to the activities of the Employer or Executive while he was employed by the Employer. The Executive specifically agrees to provide testimony and/or participate in strategy sessions with respect to litigation, claims, or investigations when requested to do so by the Employer. The Employer shall reimburse Executive for expenses associated with the same.

(b) The Employer will indemnify Executive to the fullest extent permitted by applicable laws and regulations in connection with any claims or investigations arising from his employment by the Employer and in connection with any action undertaken while he was the Chief Executive Officer of or acting at the behest or on behalf of the Employer and within the scope of his employment. This will include advancing the costs of defense incurred by Executive to the extent permitted by the laws of the State of _____, provided that the Employer approves Executive's counsel and Executive is party to any joint defense agreement that the Employer may propose.

(c) The Employer agrees to continue to cover Executive under its director's and officer's and other liability insurance (to the extent permitted by said insurance policy) and to provide a defense to him against all costs, charges, and expenses incurred in connection with any action, suit, or proceeding to which he may be made a party by reasons of his duties as Chief Executive Officer of the Employer or for services requested by the Employer under this Agreement.

10. <u>No Representations</u>.

This document constitutes the final, complete, and exclusive statement of the terms of the agreement among all the parties to this Agreement relating to the rights granted by it and the obligations assumed under it. No party has been induced to enter into this Agreement by, nor has any party relied on, any representation or warranty outside those expressly set forth in this Agreement. This Agreement may be supplemented, amended, or modified only by the mutual agreement of the parties, in writing signed by all the parties. If a court or an arbitrator of competent jurisdiction holds any provision of this Agreement to be illegal, unenforceable, or invalid in whole or in part for any reason, the validity and enforceability of the remaining provisions, or portions of them, will not be affected.

11. <u>Successors</u>.

All of the terms and provisions contained in this Agreement shall inure to the benefit of and shall be binding upon the parties hereto and their respective heirs, legal representatives, successors, and assigns.

12. <u>Severability and Governing Law</u>.

(a) With the exception of Section 8(a) and (b), should any of the provisions in this Agreement be declared or be determined to be illegal or invalid, all remaining parts, terms, or provisions shall be valid, and the illegal or invalid part, term, or provision shall be deemed not to be a part of this Agreement.

(b) This Agreement is made and entered into in the State of _____ and shall in all respects be interpreted, enforced, and governed under the laws of _____. Venue for resolution of disputes shall be in [<u>county</u>], [<u>state</u>].

13. <u>Proper Construction</u>.

(a) The language of all parts of this Agreement shall in all cases be construed as a whole according to its fair meaning, and not strictly for or against any of the parties.

(b) As used in this Agreement, the term "or" shall be deemed to include the term "and/or" and the singular or plural number shall be deemed to include the other whenever the context so indicates or requires.

(c) The paragraph headings used in this Agreement are intended solely for convenience of reference and shall not in any manner amplify, limit, modify, or otherwise be used in the interpretation of any of the provisions hereof.

14. Understanding of Consequences.

(a) The parties have been advised by counsel and understand and acknowledge the significance and consequence of the specific intention to release all claims and thereby assume full responsibility for any injuries, damages, losses, or liability that they may hereafter incur.

(b) Executive further certifies that he has read the terms of this Agreement, including the Releases in Section 8, and has had an opportunity to review this Agreement with his attorney, and that he understands its terms and effects. Executive further acknowledges that he is executing this Agreement voluntarily, with a full understanding of its terms and effects, in exchange for consideration which he acknowledges is adequate and satisfactory to him. Executive further represents and warrants that he has been informed that he has up to twenty-one (21) days to review this Agreement before signing it and that he may revoke all parts of this Agreement within twenty-one (21) days of signing it by informing the Employer of such revocation in writing on or before the seventh day. If Executive exercises his option to revoke this Agreement, this Agreement shall be entirely null and void.

15. Counterparts; Execution.

This Agreement may be executed in one or more counterparts, and by the different parties hereto in separate counterparts, each of which when executed shall be deemed to be an original, but all of which taken together shall constitute one and the same agreement. This Agreement may be executed by facsimile.

IN WITNESS WHEREOF, the parties have caused this Agreement to be executed on the date written below.

EMPLOYER

WITNESS: BY:

[Name/Title]

DATE:

WITNESS:

DATE:

[Name of Executive]

EXHIBIT A

Benefits Continued During Severance Period

The following benefits shall be continued during the time that Executive receives severance pay in accordance with Section 2(b) of the Separation Agreement:

References

Alexander, J. 1999. *The Changing Character of Hospital Governance.* Chicago: The Health Research and Educational Trust.

Alexander, J., B. Weiner, R. Bogue, and J. Isaacs. 1999. *Hospital Governance Trends.* Unpublished manuscript.

Alexander, J. A., M. L. Fennell, and M. T. Halpern. 1993. "Leadership Instability in Hospitals: The Influence of Board–CEO Relations and Organizational Growth and Decline." *Administrative Science Quarterly* 38: 92–93.

American College of Healthcare Executives. 2008a. "CEO's, Attitudes About Contracts for Themselves and Their Management Teams." CEO Circle White Paper. Chicago: ACHE.

———. 2008b. "Evaluating the Performance of the Hospital or Health System CEO," Professional Policy Statement. [Online information.] www.ache.org/policy/ceo-perf.cfm.

———. 2008c. "Key Industry Facts: 2008." Insert. *Healthcare Executive* 23 (5).

———. 2008d. "Terms of Employment for Healthcare Executives," Professional Policy Statement. [Online information.] www.ache.org/policy/employmt.cfm.

———. 2008e. "Top Issues Confronting Hospitals: 2007." *Healthcare Executive* 23 (2): 84–85.

———. 2007. "Executive Employment Contracts and Performance Evaluations." CEO Circle White Paper. Chicago: ACHE.

———. 2006. "CEO Fax Survey on Executive Employment Contracts and CEO Evaluation." Chicago: ACHE.

———. 2004. *Evaluating the Performance of the Hospital CEO.* Chicago: ACHE.

———. 1999. "CEO Circle Fax Survey." *CEO Circle Newsletter.* Chicago: ACHE.

———. 1938. *Contracts of Hospital Administrators with Suggestions as to Form.* Report of the Model Contracts Committee, Dallas, Texas, September 26.

American College of Healthcare Executives and American Hospital Association. 1993. *Evaluating the Performance of the Hospital CEO in a Total Quality Management Environment.* Chicago: ACHE.

American College of Healthcare Executives, American Hospital Association, American Medical Association, and Ernst & Young. 1993. *The Partnership Study: A Study of the Roles and Working Relationships of the Hospital Board Chairman, CEO, and Medical Staff President.* Chicago: ACHE.

American College of Hospital Administrators. 1985. Membership Advancement Study. Unpublished data. Chicago: ACHA.

———. 1984. *The Evolving Role of the Hospital Chief Executive Officer.* Chicago: ACHA.

———. 1982. *Contracts for Hospital Chief Executive Officers.* Chicago: ACHA.

American Hospital Association, American Society for Health Care Human Resources Administration, Healthcare Financial Management Association, and Ernst & Young LLP. 1994. *Executive Benefits Survey.* Atlanta: Ernst & Young LLP.

Arrick, M. D. 2008. "Finance: Nonprofit Performance Peaking amid Growing Headwinds." In *Futurescan 2008: Healthcare Trends and Implications 2008–2013,* 10–14. Chicago: Health Administration Press.

Becker, C. 2008. "Nowhere to Run, or Hide." *Modern Healthcare* 38 (16): 6–7.

Bogue, R. J., J. C. Isaacs, F. Abbey, and A. Hagel. 1997. *Shining Light on Your Board's Passage to the Future.* Chicago: American Hospital Association and Ernst & Young, LLP.

Boys, C. 1986. Interview with author, September.

Business Wire. 2007. "United Healthcare and Advocate Health Care Sign New Long-Term Agreement." *Business Wire,* November 21.

Capell, P. 2008. "Terminated? Who Cares?" *Wall Street Journal,* April 14: R4.

Challenger, J. 2008. Personal correspondence, February.

Christoforo, J. A. 2000. Interview with author, October.

Cohen, K. R. 2008. *Best Practices for Developing Effective and Enduring Board/CEO Relationships.* Chicago: American Hospital Association.

Cotter, T. 2009. Personal correspondence, March.

———. 2008a. Personal correspondence, May.

———. 2008b. Interview with author, February.

———. 2001. Interview with author, April.

Culver, J. P., III. 1986. Interview with author, September.

Currier, E. 1986. Interview with author, September.

Dye, C. 2008. Interview with author, February 28.

———. 2001. Interview with author, April.

Evans, M. 2008a. "New 990 Gets Down to Specifics."*Modern Healthcare*, April 14: 14.

———. 2008b. "Still Worried About Money." *Modern Healthcare*, January 7: 8.

Evans, M., and V. Galloro. 2008. "M&A Trend: No Big Deal: Tight Credit Could Make It Tougher to Finance Large For-Profit Acquisitions Like Those That Made the Headlines the Past Two Years." *Modern Healthcare*, January 21: 21.

Fisher, M. 1984. "Contractually Speaking." *Forbes*. February 13: 150–154.

Ford, D. 2008. Interview with author, September.

———. 2001. Interview with author, April.

Franck, R. 2000. Interview with author, April.

Independent Sector. 2002. "What You Need to Know about the Proposed IRS Regulations." [Online article; retrieved 9/9/08.] www.independentsector.org/PDFs/sanctions.pdf.

Institute of Medicine. 2008. *To Err Is Human: Building a Safer Health System.* [Online information; retrieved 9/10/08.] www.iom.edu/Object.File/Master/4/117/ToErr-8pager.pdf.

Integrated Healthcare Strategies. 2007. *2007 Compensation Survey.* Minneapolis, MN: Integrated Health Strategies.

Irving Levin Associates. 2009. "Third Quarter Health Care M&A Bucks Market Meltdown." [Online article, retrieved 2/12/09.] www.levinassociates.com/pressroom/pressreleases/pr2008/pr810mamq3.htm.

Johnson, J. G. 1994. Interview with author, June.

Kastel, G. 2008. "Tax Exempt Organizations Should Begin Assessing Redesigned Form 990." [Online article; retrieved 9/23/08.] www.faegre.com/showarticle.aspx?Show=5501.

Kaufman, N. S. 2008. "Physicians: Employment Reemerges as Strategy to Align Incentives." In *Futurescan 2008: Healthcare Trends and Implications 2008–2013*, 30. Chicago: Health Administration Press.

Khaliq, A., D. Thompson, and S. Walston. 2006. "Perceptions of Hospital CEOs About the Effects of CEO Turnover," *Hospital Topics* 84 (4): 21–27.

Knowles, F. 2003. "Advocate Set to End Ties with United Healthcare." *Chicago Sun-Times*, September 15.

Kopman, A. 1994. Interview with author, June.

Lee Hecht Harrison. 2005. *Severance and Separation Benefits: Benchmarks for Evaluating Your Policies.* Woodcliff Lake, NJ: Lee Hecht Harrison.

Malaney, S. C. 2001. Interview with author, May.

Miller, S. T. 2001. *Rebuttable Presumption Procedure Is Key to Easy Intermediate Sanctions Compliance.* [Online information; retrieved 9/9/08.] www.irs.gov/pub/irs-utl/m4958a2.pdf.

Minow, N. 1999. "Company Response Report—CEO Contracts." [Online article; retrieved 9/28/00.] www.thecorporatelibrary.com/CEOs.

Modern Healthcare. 2005. "By the Numbers." Supplement. *Modern Healthcare* 35: 12.

Morand, P. G. 1994. Interview with author, July.

Mulholland, D. M., III. 1994. Personal correspondence, September.

Nadler, D. 1964. "Organizational Frame Bending: Types of Change in the Complex Organization." In *Corporate Transformation*, edited by R. Kilman and T. J. Covin, 79. San Francisco: Jossey-Bass.

Name withheld by request. 1986. Interview with author, September.

Notebaert, E. 1986. Interview with author, September.

Nye, D. 1988. "Trust Is a Well-Drawn Employment Contract." *Across the Board* 25 (10): 32.

Ollier Weber, D. 2006. "Friction Points." *Physician Executive,* July–August: 9.

Patricia, S., A. S. Bacon, and F. G. Carter. 1935. *The Hospital Administrator: An Analysis of His Duties, Responsibilities, Relationships and Obligations.* Chicago: Physicians Record Company.

Prybil, L., S. Levey, R. Peterson, D. Heinrich, P. Brezinski, J. Price, G. Zamba, and W. Roach. 2008. "Governance in Nonprofit Community Health Systems: An Initial Report on CEO Perspectives," [Online article; retrieved 9/22/08.] www.public-health.uiowa.edu/news/pdf/021508-release.pdf.

Schaeffer, B. E. 1989. "The Employment Contract as a Recruitment and Retention Tool." In *The Hay Group Guide to Executive Compensation*, edited by T. J. Flannery, 141. Chicago: Pluribus Press.

Schoenberger. M. 2009. Personal correspondence, March.

Schlosser, J. 2008. Interview with author, February.

———. 2001. Interview with author, April.

Steiger, A. 1994. Interview with author, August.

Sullivan, Cotter and Associates, Inc. 2008. *2008 Survey of Manager and Executive Compensation in Hospitals and Health Systems*. Detroit, MI: Sullivan, Cotter and Associates, Inc.

Tarrant, J. 1985. *Perks and Parachutes: Negotiating Your Executive Employment Contract*. New York: Simon and Schuster.

Thomas, P. 1986. Interview with author, September.

Tyler, J. L. 2008a. Personal correspondence, October,

———. 2008b. Interview with author, September.

———. 2002. *Tyler's Guide: The Health Care Executive's Job Search*, 3rd ed. Chicago: Health Administration Press.

———. 2000. Interview with author, April.

———. 1994. Interview with author, September.

Vesely, R. 2008a. "Ain't No Sunshine. . . ." *Modern Healthcare*, July 7: 17.

———. 2008b. "Providers Getting Out: Systems Selling Managed-Care Businesses." *Modern Healthcare*, April 21: 10.

Wegmiller, D. C. 2001a. Interview with author, May.

———. 2001b. Interview with author, April.

Weil, P. A., and D. M. Mulholland, III. 1989. "Executive Contracts: From the Organization's and Candidate's Perspectives." In *The Health Care Executive Search: A Guide to Recruiting and Job Seeking*, edited by E. A. Simendinger and T. F. Moore, 72–75. Rockville, MD: Aspen Publishers, Inc.

Wendling, J. T. 1994. Interview with author, July.

Index

About the Principal Author

Dr. Reed L. Morton, FACHE, is director of the Healthcare Executive Career Resource Center at the American College of Healthcare Executives (ACHE). Morton's healthcare career has been multi-faceted. He has held teaching and administrative appointments at the Universities of Iowa, Michigan, Chicago, and Notre Dame, and has directed health planning with public agencies and private health systems. He has authored articles on healthcare marketing, governance and leadership, and career development.

Dr. Morton joined the ACHE staff in 1987 to head the Hospital Leadership Project. Subsequent assignments included coordinating the Carolinas Healthcare Leadership Demonstration Project and several task forces on career development. Morton is a past president of the Chicago Health Executives Forum and served on the boards of the healthcare division of the Academy of Management and the Administrative Fellowship Coordinating Council. He is a member of the Association of Career Professionals International and serves as a reviewer for a number of healthcare-related journals.

Sample Contracts on CD-ROM

This book includes a CD-ROM of the sample contracts and letters of agreement presented in appendixes D through G. These documents can be edited using Microsoft Word or a compatible word-processing program.

Please keep in mind that these documents are only models. They are intended to serve as guides for negotiation between the executive and the organization. The details of your final contract will depend on the institution's situation, the needs and desires of the executive and the board, and the laws of the state in which the institution is located. As with any contractual arrangement, the advice of legal, financial, and benefits consultants should be sought before finalizing the agreement.

PC USERS

If you are using a PC, simply insert the CD-ROM into your computer's CD drive. A menu including links to each of the sample contracts and letters will load automatically.

MAC USERS

If you are using a Mac, insert the CD-ROM into your computer's CD-ROM drive and click on the **Sample Contracts** icon that appears on your desktop. Click on the folder named **Mac**. This folder contains the sample contracts and letters.